GW00537096

LOUISE BROWN

My life as the...
WORLD'S FIRST
TEST-TUBE BABY

Written and researched by Martin Powell

BRISTOL BOOKS CIC

Bristol Books CIC, 1 Lyons Court, Long Ashton Business Park,
Yanley Lane, Long Ashton, Bristol BS41 9LB

Louise Brown: My life as the world's first test-tube baby,
written and researched by Martin Powell

Published by Bristol Books 2015

ISBN: 978-1-909446-08-3

Copyright: Bristol Books CIC

Design: Joe Burt (joe@wildsparkdesign.com)
Cover photography: Neil Phillips

Martin Powell has asserted his right under the Copyright, Designs and Patents Act
of 1988 to be identified as the author of this work.

All rights reserved. This book may not be reproduced or transmitted in any form
or in any means without the prior written consent of the publisher, except by a
reviewer who wishes to quote brief passages in connection with a review written in
a newspaper or magazine or broadcast on television, radio or on the internet.

A CIP record for this book is available from the British Library.

The author and publisher have made every effort to ensure that the information in this book was correct
at the time of going to press and all permissions have been sought for images and information used.
Any errors or admissions are unintentional. This autobiography is based on the memories
of those who were at the events in question and as such are a partial account of events.
The publishers are happy to correct factual errors in future editions.

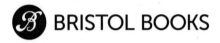 BRISTOL BOOKS

Bristol Books CIC is a not-for-profit Community Interest Company
that publishes important and untold stories about lives,
communities, places and events of significance and interest

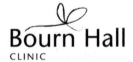
Bourn Hall
CLINIC

First Edition hardback produced
in association with Bourn Hall Clinic

This book is dedicated to:

Lesley Brown, John Brown,
Patrick Steptoe and Robert Edwards

The four people who made me and changed the world

CONTENTS

PROLOGUE

The people involved in my birth were true pioneers. My story wouldn't exist without them. Firstly there was my Mum and Dad – Lesley Brown and John Gilbert Brown from Bristol. They wanted to have a baby but couldn't conceive naturally.

They heard of the work of Patrick Steptoe, obstetrician and gynaecologist and Robert Edwards, biologist and physiologist who were developing methods to help people conceive. Helped by Jean Purdy, research assistant and qualified nurse, the two men had a small laboratory in a cottage hospital called Kershaw's near Oldham, Lancashire.

Mum on July 25, 1978 was the first woman to successfully have a baby as a result of their technique – now known worldwide as IVF (in-vitro fertilisation). This is the story of my life as a world first.

Chapter 1

"NORMAL" BABY

J ust about the one thing that everybody seems to know about me is that I was born! Hardly a television or pub quiz goes by without a question about me. Usually it is "What was the name of the world's first test-tube baby?" Sometimes it is turned around to "What was special about baby Louise Brown born on July 25, 1978?" and once or twice I have heard the question: "What was the middle name of Louise Brown, the world's first test-tube baby?"

I don't suppose there are many people that can say they were world famous within hours of being born - but my name made headlines in just about every country in the world.

Of course the people who really deserved the headlines were the wonderful scientist Dr. Robert Edwards and the gynaecologist Patrick Steptoe, who had worked for years on medical techniques in a bid to help women who couldn't have children to experience the joy of being parents.

Women like my Mum, Lesley, who along with my Dad, John had spent 10 years trying to have a baby and had been told categorically by doctors that there was no hope. By pure chance they became pioneers when they grabbed at one small opportunity given to them by the experimental programme of Robert Edwards and Patrick Steptoe and so booked themselves a place in history.

Not many people born in the 1970s can see a video of their birth. Not only is there a full colour film of every second of my first moments in life but now it is posted on YouTube for the world to see.

These days with video cameras on everybody's phone it is not that unusual but for that to happen at my birth, discussions had to be held between the Minister for Health and the Regional Health Authority in Oldham, Lancashire to enable the cine camera to be allowed in to the delivery room. In fact it was only a few minutes before my birth that a contract was signed to enable the filming to go ahead and Patrick Steptoe and Robert Edwards had to get tough with the authorities, threatening to go ahead with the birth without the cameras present.

Of course they knew it was vital to have the birth on film to prove that they had achieved something, which up until then had been impossible. They had created a new human life - me - in a glass petri dish then successfully transplanted the embryo back into my mother for a normal pregnancy and birth. "In Vitro" simply means "in glass" and what they had done was come up with a new way of creating babies - now known as IVF - In Vitro Fertilisation.

Yes, despite those last minute rows Robert Edwards, who my family always called Bob, and Patrick Steptoe really wanted that film to be made. It would provide proof of what they had done. Proof that they had finally achieved something that they had worked on for many years.

Patrick Steptoe had been told as a medical student that two per cent of women could not have babies because of blocked fallopian tubes. As a gynaecologist he had looked at ways tubes could be unblocked and eventually at how eggs could be removed and put back into the womb on the other side of the blockage so that a baby could result.

Bob Edwards, as a student in Edinburgh in the 1950s had seen how fertilised eggs had been removed from a mouse and put into a different mouse and had grown quite successfully in the womb. The two men met in 1968 and their determination to help women with blocked fallopian tubes to have babies resulted in my birth 10 years later.

Thanks to that film I can honestly say exactly what my birth was like. Mum needed to have a cesarean so was given the anaesthetic by senior anaesthetist Dr. Finlay Campbell in a room at exactly 11.31pm. These days women can remain conscious during a cesarean delivery but in 1978 it meant for Mum that she would be totally out of it and so not have any memory of the birth of her first baby.

Just seven minutes later she was wheeled into the operating theatre. On the film she looks like something out of one of those Roswell alien incidents! She is lying scarily still on the trolley as it is wheeled into the theatre. She is then lifted from the trolley on to an operating table.

People are busying themselves about and another man from the Central Office of Information - the Government press office - is hanging about with a stills camera in full hospital scrubs.

Patrick Steptoe gave a little commentary for the sake of the camera as he and his team prepared to bring me into the world.

"This is Mrs. Lesley Brown. She is now 38 weeks pregnant and she's had persistent toxemia." He is handed a green cloth that he unfolds to place over my mum's bare abdomen. "All our tests have shown that the growth of the baby is satisfactory and that it's mature."

He then introduces the others gathered around: "My anaesthetist is Dr. Finlay Campbell, Dr. John Webster assisting. My theatre sister is Sister Astell."

Edith Astell was in fact one of two "Ediths" in the room. To the right of Steptoe stood Edith Marshall, scrubbed and gowned and wearing gloves. Her job was to be handed me the second I was born. A theatre nurse called Jennifer Thompson had the job of sterilising and preparing all the medical instruments. Apparently there was also a full back-up team of pediatric specialists nearby ready to be called in if anything went wrong.

Mr. Steptoe made the incisions and wrestled my head out skillfully and one of the women around the operating table says "girl". Then

Patrick Steptoe says: "It's a girl, as was expected." While he is saying that Edith Marshall puts a tube into my throat to prompt my breathing.

Patrick Steptoe said: "The baby's in pretty good condition at birth. You can now hand it to our..." I interrupted him with my first cry and someone notes that I made that first noise at just 20 seconds old. Most of my family and friends would say that I haven't really shut up since!

Patrick Steptoe's own notes soon after the birth put the time that he pulled me through the "letter box opening" he had made at 11.47pm.

He said in an account of the birth published in 1980 (A Matter of Life) about that moment: "Glorious. She was chubby, full of muscular tone. The cord was pulsating strongly although it was hooked around the left thigh. I held the head low and we sucked and cleared the mouth and throat. She took a deep breath. Then she yelled and yelled and yelled. I laid her down, all pink and furious, and saw at once that she was externally perfect and beautiful.

"One minute after the birth the cord stopped pulsating and we clamped it, divided it, and handed the baby to Edith Marshall.

"The new citizen continued to cry very loudly, and how we all loved that wonderful sound."

Because I was the first baby ever to have been conceived through IVF they wanted to check everything about me and a few medical checks are made before - still screaming - they placed me in an incubator and someone says: "The baby is perfectly normal".

What the film doesn't show is the full range of checks and prodding and probing that went on to ensure that there was nothing at all abnormal about the baby that had been conceived in the most unusual way. Those checks were carried out by a Dr. Don Hilson, who had been part of the standby squad in case something went wrong. I had weighed in at 5lb 12oz.

Dr. Hilson and his team carried out more than 60 different tests on me and his attitude in my first hours and days of life upset Mum. She never had anything but praise for Bob Edwards and Patrick Steptoe, who never forgot that Mum was a human being and I was a little baby.

Dr. Hilson on the other hand was a little more matter-of-fact in his approach as far as Mum was concerned and Mum got upset at his constant "tests" to check every aspect of her new baby. John Webster was also an essential part of the team - Mum had more time for him and affectionately called him "Dracula" because he was the one always taking blood samples from her during her pregnancy.

The film also doesn't show someone shaking my Mum awake and saying to her: "You have a beautiful baby girl". She told me how she was being brought back to consciousness while still in the operating theatre and hearing for the first time that I had been successfully born. I was held close to her but all she saw was the blurred outline of a baby before the drugs took over again and she fell back to sleep.

As she slept Dr. Hilson and his team took me away for those tests. What they were doing was basically aimed at proving to a sceptical world that creating a baby in this way did not cause any problems or abnormality. After all the tests had been carried out it was the back-up team and Dr. Hilson that declared me "normal".

It is hard to grasp now just how important that news must have been to Steptoe and Edwards. There is film of Bob Edwards coming into the operating theatre as I scream away and saying to one of the nurses: "That's a noise you are going to hear a lot of in the next few weeks." The two doctors and Jean Purdy, who had been the technical assistant when the egg and sperm had been introduced to each other nine months before in a laboratory, pose proudly holding me. For just a few moments it ceased to be a "normal" cesarean section birth and the full realisation at what the team had achieved can be seen in their eyes.

Jean Purdy was the person who first saw that the cells had divided in a laboratory in November 1977. Those cells indicated that the egg had been fertilised and it was the first sign that I was to make it into the world. Of course there was a lot to do after that. Putting the embryo back into Mum's womb and then ensuring her body didn't reject it and that the pregnancy carried on in the same way as any other normal pregnancy.

Quite what would have happened to the future of IVF if I had been born with any kind of disability or defect is hard to tell. The climate at that time was very much against the pioneers with many people saying no good could come of messing with the natural process of conception and child-birth.

The film crew were told not to film when my Dad came into the room a few minutes after I was born to see me lying in the incubator but he said he cried. He first got to hold me a little later on after going in a lift with three policemen up to the premature baby unit. They had taken me to the unit as a precaution and to protect me from the prying eyes of the world's media that were gathering outside.

It was the next morning before Mum got to see me properly for the first time. By then Edwards and Steptoe had enjoyed a nights rest and fully recovered from the operation. I was wheeled in on a trolley by Mr Steptoe himself, who handed me to Mum. I was named Louise Joy Brown - the Joy bit coming from the happiness I had brought through the circumstances of my birth.

After years of wanting to be a mother my Mum, Lesley, was unable to hold her precious bundle until later that day and when she did she found it covered in ink and bearing the marks of Dr. Hilson's checks. For some reason one of the checks he had been asked to do was to take my fingerprints. I guess they needed to check that my skin was normal.

But he left the ink on my little fingers and under my nails and that really upset Mum. Every mother will tell you just how wonderful it is to have their little perfect baby put into their arms - imagine how you would feel if the baby has already been finger-printed, probed and subjected to strange tests before you even get to give them their first cuddle.

Looking back at the way things were done in those days it seems that Mum and Dad were a bit sidelined compared to the medical team. I think that says more about the way childbirth worked generally then, rather than the particular circumstances of my birth. Fathers were hardly ever at their children's birth and certainly wouldn't have been allowed anywhere near a cesarean, which Mum had to have because of her toxemia. In 1978 the attitude was that medics knew best and any patient in a hospital was often not considered knowledgeable enough to be told what was happening to them. I think attitudes to patients and certainly to mothers and fathers have changed a great deal in my lifetime.

What I couldn't possibly know as I was screaming away - and according to all reports I did a lot of screaming in those first few weeks - was that the mere fact that I had been born was one of the most important moments in world history. My birth has been ranked alongside man walking on the moon as one of the most historic events of the 20th Century. I've learned to live with that and with the constant interest of journalists and others throughout my life.

The fact that I am "normal" has made the birth of millions of other people in the world possible - as I'm pretty sure that the pressure from those against IVF would have won the day with a lot of "I told you so" and "It's not safe" if there had been anything wrong with me.

Mum and Dad were aware that a media storm was about to break around me. Although the doctors knew that their pioneering work would grab headlines and excite interest I'm not sure they were really ready for the incredible worldwide response to what they had achieved. They were about to get hit by a firestorm of demands from television, radio, newspapers and magazines all over the world. They would also be fiercely criticised by those against what they had achieved and by the tabloid media, who just wanted a sensational story.

There is no doubt it was a sensational story. My birth had all the elements that would get a national newspaper editor excited. First of all babies are cute (even me) and everyone wants to hear a good baby story; secondly there were so many people all over the world who wanted babies but couldn't have them. My birth gave them hope and they wanted to read every word about it. If Louise Brown could be born by this technique then millions of people who believed they would never have a child might be able to have one after all.

Then there was the difficult moral and religious argument. Until I uttered that first cry nobody had ever been born by anything other than a normal conception - a man and a woman having sex and pretty much hoping for the best. Of course gynaecology had been constantly improved and various drugs and techniques had enabled babies to be born before me that in the past would not have survived. But this was different. This was a baby born without a couple having sex to make it happen - and sex sells newspapers!

That amazing combination was enough to excite the media into a frenzy. Add to that the human interest story of an ordinary working class couple willing to be the first to try a medical technique because they so much wanted a baby and the interest was incredible. On top of that one of the men responsible was called Steptoe and that was a famous name in the UK for one reason - the popular comedy *Steptoe And Son* about a rag and bone man that had been on the screens from 1962 to 1974.

The media had a lot of exciting things to chase...some were even rushing off to ask the comedians Wilfred Brambell and Harry H Corbett what they thought of my birth - just because they had played Albert and Harold Steptoe in the series - quite what they thought they could add to the debate about IVF I'm not sure.

Mum and Dad certainly didn't realise that they were opening themselves up for worldwide media interest when they embarked on the road that led to me being born. Dad had two daughters from a previous marriage, Sharon and Beverley. Beverley had been adopted and, although my Mum loved Sharon to bits and treated her like her own daughter, they were keen to have a child of their own after they had got married.

It hadn't happened for them and after going through lots of tests Mum was eventually told that it would be impossible. They thought about adoption and fostering but Mum really wanted a child of her own. Like many other couples it put a real strain on their relationship as they got increasingly desperate. I'm not sure if the marriage would have survived if they hadn't found some way to have a baby - Mum admits she got very depressed and upset and Dad found it hard to cope with that.

I suppose before going on with my story I ought to just explain a little about how my Mum and Dad ended up having a world first. They both had tough lives before suddenly becoming known all over the world.

Chapter 2

MUM AND DAD'S STORY

Mum and Dad, Lesley and John, were proud to come from Bristol in the South West of England. Even though, I suppose technically I am a Lancastrian, being born in Oldham - I really count myself as a Bristolian too. I've lived in the city all my life, just like Mum and Dad, and I love the place.

Both Mum and Dad had pretty tough upbringings in some of the roughest parts of Bristol. Mum's father walked out when she was two so she never knew him and her mother was out working or out enjoying herself in the evenings. During her childhood she never really had a proper family in the traditional sense.

Her Grandmother and Grandfather had been very good to her as a child growing up in Bristol with her brother David and it was really the times she spent with them that made her long for a proper family with a husband and children. She was very unhappy at school and was often in trouble being made to stand outside the classroom door or in the corner of the room because she was a disruptive influence.

She became too much for her Grandmother to cope with so her Mum suggested that she and her brother David find a new life in Australia. There was an emigration scheme that saw some 100,000 children go to Australia to provide labour.

Mum was shown photographs of a farm where she and David would work on the other side of the world. They were sent to a home in Kent to be assessed - but it seems Mum's naughtiness meant that she wasn't considered suitable for Australia.

It seems wicked today to think that people would send their children to the other side of the world simply because they were poor. In 2010 the then Prime Minister Gordon Brown officially apologised for the UK's role in that system and the Australian Government apologised as well - my Mum had a lucky escape.

Her Auntie Peggy took on Mum and her brother David even though she had two younger children of her own and Mum found herself in a three-bedroom house in Filton, Bristol. It wasn't an easy relationship, and reading between the lines of what I was told about those days, Mum was a real handful as a child and it must have been really difficult for Auntie Peggy to look after her.

Auntie Peggy tried to instill some discipline by being tough with her and they fell out over the chores that Auntie Peggy wanted her to do at home when she wanted to be out enjoying herself with her friends. By the time she was 11 she had started smoking and she spent most of her time with her best friend Carol. Her friends, her smoking and her lifestyle were all met with disapproval from her Auntie, who found her increasingly difficult to control. Mum wasn't doing anything really nasty, just the usual rebellious things that teenagers were doing in those post-war days that so annoyed the generation before that had been through the tough years of the 1930s and the war.

Arguments got worse at home and during one row an exasperated Peggy said: "I'm going to get you put away in a home again if you don't change your ways." Mum ran off back to her Grandmother and then stayed with her again.

As she got into her mid teens she dyed her hair platinum blonde, which was the fashion of the time and started hanging around a dive called The Holborn in central Bristol where she could get cigarettes and drink from the regulars.

Mum left school at the earliest opportunity when she was 14 and got a job in an underwear factory in Bristol.

At 15 she started going out with a mixed race lad called Frank - not only was he a bit older than her but the fact he was not white was controversial in those days in Bristol. Soon there were more rows - this time with Grandmother - over the fact she was staying out late at night and sometimes taking time off work to see Frank. That meant her money was docked so there was less money to take home to Grandmother for housekeeping.

She got the sack from her job because of her poor attendance but found a little job in a cafe and then Brooks The Cleaners where she did a manual job. Frank got into trouble and ended up in prison. Mum was angry that he had borrowed her precious transistor radio on which she listened to all the new music that was sweeping the world in the 1960s. Frank took the radio to prison and never gave it back - no teenager in the Sixties liked to be deprived of their radio and that was the end of their relationship!

By now Mum was spending more time hanging around The Holborn scrounging cigarettes – fags as she called them - from the men than she did working and that was where she met my Dad, John, who at that time was married. He was six years older than Mum.

Dad also had a difficult upbringing. He came from Knowle West, Bristol. His Mum had died of cancer when he was 10 so with his Dad and brother Keith it was a family of men. They lived in a prefab - temporary homes built in Bristol following the Second World War to replace the hundreds of homes that had been destroyed in Nazi bombing raids on the city. The family had been housed there because their home in St Dunstan's Road had been destroyed by a bomb in the Blitz of the city in 1941.

The family had been hit hard by the death of the woman in the house and Dad's Father found it tough bringing up the boys and let a few things go. Dad's Mum had been an actress and I think he inherited some of her outgoing personality because he was always the chatty one and loved socialising.

He also left school at 14 and had a series of jobs and his father took him to The Holborn where he met a woman called Margaret. By the time he was 21 Dad was married with two daughters, Sharon and Beverley.

The marriage didn't last and Dad found himself with the two young children while trying to work. Neighbours looked after the children for a short while but eventually Sharon was taken into care and Beverley was brought up by his Stepmother's daughter.

Dad found himself back with his own father and Stepmother, but things were far from happy. There were rows and one day his Stepmother threw a bowl of rice pudding at him and he left - and so was sleeping wherever he could and spending time at The Holborn drinking and that was how Mum and Dad got together.

They always told the story of how Dad walked her home to her Grandmother's house one night after she had some trouble at The Holborn with some other men. He was a familiar face to her so she called to him for help when the other men were bothering her.

He promptly told the trouble-makers where to go and then walked several miles with her to her Grandmother's house. Neither of them had the bus fare and on that walk Mum decided to leave home. Because she hadn't been working she once again didn't have the money to pay her Grandmother rent she owed. It seemed easier to walk out and be with this man, who she felt she could trust.

Dad waited in the back lane of the house while she packed her case and, leaving a note for her Grandmother, she walked out to spend her life with a man who at that time she barely knew - she was just 16. He bought her chips and they went to some railway sidings near Lawrence Hill in Bristol. They found some railway carriages. They were the old fashioned type that you see in films with compartments with a bench each side. They slept the night on the train seats - one each side of the compartment.

The two misfits had found each other and I doubt on that first night sleeping in a railway siding they could imagine that they were to be together for half a century and make world history. Mum always said that from day one she knew she could trust Dad.

After a few weeks John and Lesley were found by a railway employee sleeping on the train and evicted from their temporary home. For a while both were out of work, spending their days drinking cider and blackcurrant at The Three Tuns pub in Bristol and drifting around. Somehow they scraped enough money together for a rented room in a house in St Paul's, an area mostly populated by the West Indian immigrant community that was establishing itself in Bristol.

The pair were living on means-tested benefits and fell into a routine where they would leave the rented room in the morning - Mum usually nicking a spoonful of the West Indian landlord's condensed milk as she left to eat as her breakfast. They would walk down by The Cut in Bristol, which in warm weather had a terrible smell because in those days sewage still discharged into the river. They would be first in the pub when it opened, drink heavily all day, then laze around until they could go back to their room.

Thankfully they broke out of the destructive lifestyle when Dad managed to get a job as a bus conductor. He had a series of jobs but eventually ended up working on the railways for 21 years.

After Dad got a job they moved to City Road, St Paul's where they rented a basement flat and they wanted to look after Dad's daughters. Beverley was happy where she was and Dad had fallen out with his Stepmother's family, but they hatched a plan to get Sharon out of care. Sharon had been taken into care aged 18 months old and was in a children's home in Fishponds. They went to visit her and Mum got on well with the "skinny little girl". She knitted her some clothes and they started visiting regularly.

Amazingly they managed to get her released from the home just by ringing from a nearby phone box and saying that Dad was back with his wife. The authorities didn't question them and Sharon, now aged three, went to live with Mum and Dad and was brought up by Mum.

They were a family at last, although for a while they couldn't get married because Dad was still married to his first wife. After six years the divorce came through and they were married at Bristol Register Office.

They wanted to have a child that came from both of them but Mum never seemed to get pregnant. Soon she sensed something was wrong.

Mum had all sorts of tests to work out why she couldn't get pregnant. They tried for 10 years with no luck after getting married. They were told that they had no chance of ever having a baby. Mum became depressed as the years went by. She had an operation at Bristol Royal Infirmary to try to unblock her tubes but it was no use.

With Dad in regular work, although not brilliantly paid and Mum able to do some jobs as well as look after Sharon they became more of a regular couple and got a small house at 4 Hassell Drive in Newtown, St Philip's, Bristol.

It wasn't much by most people's standards but for a couple who had started out squatting in a railway carriage it was quite a responsibility. It was right in the centre of Bristol so close to the railway lines. By now Dad was working as a lorry driver for the railway company British Rail.

Mum thought that once she was more settled in a home she might conceive - but it made no difference. During another trip to the doctor about her depression it was suggested she might seek expert help.

Bristol Central Health Clinic in Tower Hill is the place where anyone with any kind of infertility problem in Bristol is sent and Mum was referred to the clinic by her doctor, who I think was just trying to give her a bit of hope because of her depression, which the doctor believed had been brought on because she was unable to have a baby of her own. Mum and Dad were told to write to the medical officer at the clinic, Dr. Rosalin Hinton, to see if there was any way that they could conceive a child. She wrote to her in the summer of 1976 and in June Dr. Hinton wrote back. The letter was the start of a long journey.

It read: "Thank you for your letter. I shall of course be pleased to see you and your husband and can offer you an appointment on Thursday 6 July at 10.45am. However, after an operation such as yours, obviously you must realise that the chances of anything being done are not very great."

With hardly any reason for optimism they went to see Dr. Hinton. Mum underwent lots of painful tests and Dr. Hinton confirmed there was no hope of a baby. The tests showed that Mum's blocked fallopian tubes were inoperable. The previous attempt to unblock the tubes just hadn't worked and nothing more could be done.

But Dr. Hinton had heard about the work of Patrick Steptoe in Oldham. He was asking for patients with blocked fallopian tubes. It was experimental work and Dr. Hinton told Mum that the treatment sounded like "science fiction" and was only a "million to one chance" of being successful. But as far as Mum and Dad were concerned it kept their hope alive so they asked for their details to be sent to him with a referral from Dr. Hinton.

Mum didn't really understand or take in what Dr. Hinton told her. She heard that Patrick Steptoe had carried out treatments on wealthy private patients and she simply thought he had a technique that might just work. It wasn't until she was well into her pregnancy that she twigged that the technique had never been successfully carried out before.

In Autumn 1976 Patrick Steptoe got a letter from Dr. Hinton outlining my Mum's history, which included the operation at the Bristol Royal Infirmary in 1970 to try to get the tubes unblocked. Although that operation had failed Patrick Steptoe could see that Mum was still likely to be producing eggs that could be captured. Dad had already fathered Sharon and Beverley so didn't appear to have any problems. Patrick Steptoe's idea was to take an egg from Mum and in a glass petri dish introduce it to sperm from my Dad. He would then carefully wait for the cells to split. The idea was to then plant it back into my Mum's womb for a routine pregnancy after that.

Bob Edwards had the scientific knowledge to do all the laboratory work and had been working with Patrick Steptoe, who was the expert on how women's bodies work. Soon Mum and Dad were invited to Oldham for an interview. Part of that interview it seems was to judge their character and how much they really wanted the baby.

Mum's first news of this was another letter from Dr. Hinton on September 26, 1976. This one said simply: "This is to let you know that I have heard from Mr. Steptoe that he is willing to see you to discuss the chances of his treating you. I have asked him to send you an appointment direct. It will be at St John Street, Manchester. You should be hearing from him shortly. Best wishes and good luck."

It had been just 10 days since Dr. Hinton had confirmed that she was contacting Steptoe. The next thing that happened was that a little card arrived. It said "Mr. P. C Steptoe presents his compliments and suggests you see him by appointment on Wednesday November 10, 1976 at 3.15pm at 18 John Street Manchester, M3 4DQ".

The date and time had been typed on to a pre-printed appointment card. Mum and Dad had some hope - there was just the small matter of getting to a Wednesday afternoon appointment over 180 miles away!

Mum said that from the moment she met Patrick Steptoe she felt she could trust him. Although he was abrupt and professional she never had any doubt that he would help her get pregnant. He explained that before Mum could have the IVF treatment she would have to have a laparoscopy to see what the effects of the previous operation had been and whether it was possible to get to the eggs in her ovaries.

Patrick Steptoe wrote that Dad was very protective of Mum and would not want many risks taken. He said of Mum: "She was quietly determined, strong in resolve, unlikely to panic, and would suffer whatever was necessary with stoicism" - a pretty good summary of my Mum from just one meeting!

By February 1977 Mum was back in Oldham for the diagnostic laparoscopy, which was carried out on February 26. As far as Mum was concerned it wasn't good news. Steptoe told her that it was not possible to get an egg from her left ovaries without an operation being carried out. That operation would cost money that they just didn't have.

In early summer 1977 Mum, Dad and Sharon went on a short holiday in a caravan and when they came back a cheque for £800 was waiting for them - Dad had won the football pools and they could afford the operation!

Patrick Steptoe carried out a laparotomy on Mum on August 8, 1977 - that operation establishes that it was at least possible to collect eggs from Mum. But that had to be done at the precise time of the month.

I'm probably doing a great disservice to all the science that went into the process. Fluids had to be just right, special instruments invented for the first time and there was always the idea that this wasn't quite morally right - or even possible - that was put about by some others in the medical profession. Steptoe and Edwards fought these battles and Mum was just one of a number of ladies that they were treating at Kershaw's Cottage Hospital in Oldham where they had set up a pioneering clinic.

In fact another woman who she met during treatment fell pregnant and seemed to be on course to be the first - but sadly there was a problem in the pregnancy and she lost the baby. It was pure chance that Mum happened to be the one lying on that operating table on July 25, 1978 and that I was the first successful baby conceived in this way.

After one part of the procedure Mum and Dad travelled back to Bristol on the train as they couldn't afford to stay in Oldham overnight. Her stitches came apart and she spent most of the journey trying to stop blood spreading across her clothes.

With the programme being carried out almost 180 miles away from home there was a lot of travelling for Mum and Dad and, more importantly it meant that when I was born they were a long way from their friends and family.

Mum stayed in Oldham for weeks and met other women who were having the same treatment. As each of the women was told the treatment had not worked and went home without a baby she cried at their sadness. It was on November 10, 1977 at 11am that Mum had the operation to remove the egg - Dad had also been asked to produce a fresh semen specimen.

Before Mum was awake the team had mixed the egg and the sperm together. Mum's first question when she came around from the op to Steptoe was "Did you get an egg?" He replied: "Yes, a very nice egg. You can go back to sleep."

Now it was over to Bob Edwards and his team. It was Jean Purdy looking through the microscope that evening who noted that fertilisation of the egg had taken place and a two-cell embryo was recorded. Once the embryo had divided into eight cells Mum was prepared for the tricky procedure of putting the fertilised egg into her womb. That completed, she returned to Bristol with Dad just hoping that the whole procedure would be successful - unlike the other ladies she had met.

In early December 1977 Mum had gone into the Broadmead shopping centre in town to do some Christmas shopping with Sharon. The parcels and packages piled up and she walked around the shopping centre laden with bags before making her way home on the bus and carrying the heavy bags back home. In the post that day was a little envelope postmarked Oldham. Dad was at home so he opened it up to find the letter from Bob Edwards. It read:

"Just a short note to let you know that the early results on your blood and urine samples are very encouraging, and indicate that you might be in early pregnancy.

"So please take things quietly - no skiing, climbing or anything too strenuous including Xmas shopping!

"If you should wish to get in touch with me for any reason before seeing Mr Steptoe next week, my laboratory number is --- and my home number is ---, Best wishes."

Dad anxiously waited and when Mum arrived laden with bags of festive shopping he admonished her for carrying so much - one of the things the note asked her not to do! The pair of them were astonished and just kept reading that note over and over again. Mum kept it in her wardrobe forever.

Mum only had one alcoholic drink while she was pregnant with me - a sherry on Christmas Day 1977 - but it made her sick and she was so worried that she might lose the baby that she didn't drink anything else until after I was born.

She smoked all the way through the pregnancy though, secretly puffing cigarettes out of the window of the toilets at the hospital in Oldham in the later stages of pregnancy for fear of angering the doctors.

Mum had little contact with Bob Edwards once she was pregnant as Patrick Steptoe took over. Bob Edwards made friends with Dad and during the last few weeks of pregnancy was there to support him. As he was not a medical doctor he didn't examine Mum but he came in to see her on a number of occasions as the pregnancy progressed. He was always in a rush travelling from Cambridge, where he had his laboratories, to Oldham and Mum was amused at the fact that he wore sandals in all weathers.

There were many trips to Oldham to be endured over the next few months as every stage of the pregnancy had to be checked.

The first realisation that my birth would excite major press interest happened in April before I was born. The New York Post had written a story saying there were "on-going pregnancies" as a result of the pioneering and sensational work of Edwards and Steptoe. That sparked a story in the Oldham newspaper - and one report on April 20 said that the first test-tube baby would be born in Oldham in July and that the parents had been offered £100,000 for the exclusive rights to the story.

The reports of vast amounts of money were pure speculation by newspapers that felt that the story was being kept from them. In their minds that could only be because some other media organisation had got an "exclusive".

The truth was my birth was still three months away and although the doctors were pleased with Mum's progress through the pregnancy they had no idea whether it would continue that way. All the way through the pregnancy the doctors reported that the growth of the baby inside Mum was slow and - as they were breaking new ground - they could never be complacent or confident that I would be born. In fact Mum and Dad were only just realising quite how significant the birth would be. Although they had been told it was experimental and ground-breaking Mum thought other babies must have been born by this method and it was the interest of the media that finally made it dawn on her that this was going to be a very different baby!

Most of the reporters were poking their noses around Oldham trying to find out information.

The trips from Bristol to Oldham and back got tougher as the pregnancy progressed and then one day just after Mum had returned from Oldham there was a knock on the door at home and it was a reporter from the Sun newspaper. By chance Dad had dropped in during the working day to check on Mum. Dad answered the door to him and that was the first time he heard the phrase "test-tube baby".

Mum had been knitting baby clothes when the doorbell went and had heard the brief conversation between the reporter - who gave his name as Charles Garside, and Dad. Dad told the reporter: "You seem to know more about it than I do mate." And in many ways he probably did!

Dad shut the door telling the reporter: "You've got the wrong place." Worried about leaving Mum on her own he sneaked Mum out through the back door to stay at my Uncle David's house for a few days.

Charles Garside kept popping up and writing letters trying to collar Dad. On April 27 he wrote Dad a little letter. It said: "Dear Mr Brown, We can't go on meeting like this! All I wanted to ask you this morning was whether or not you had received my first letter. I also wanted to draw your attention to the enclosed article from yesterday's Daily Mail as an indication of the amount of interest in this story.

"As I said in my previous note I only want to get you to listen to what I have to say. My paper would like an interview with you and

Lesley about your hopes and feelings at this time.

"You have my absolute assurance that you would NOT be named or identified in any way. In return we would reward you with a substantial financial payment which perhaps you would like to use as a deposit for a house of your own or for whatever purpose you decide.

"I beg you listen at least to what I have to say. If you are still uncertain then perhaps I could meet your father or father in law whenever or wherever you like and they could pass the details on.

"I am now staying at the Holiday Inn, Bristol. If you or a relative could ring me this evening at 7.30pm or later at your convenience I would be happy to come and outline my proposals. The last thing I want is to cause distress for you or your family so you have nothing to fear or to lose by listening to what I have to say."

It was the first mention of money being paid by the press. The words "cheque-book journalism" would soon mean something to Mum and Dad. For now they were keeping their heads down, not even confirming they were the couple involved and just hoping the pregnancy continued well.

Dad had more idea about the worldwide interest in the birth than Mum. Bob Edwards had filled him in on just how significant my birth would be and the reaction that was likely to take place around the world. They decided not to tell Mum too much as they didn't want to cause her stress during her pregnancy.

There is no doubt that it was much more of a man's world in 1978 and it was Dad and Bob Edwards who did the eventual deals with the media without really ever consulting Mum about it.

The second time Mum realised how significant the birth would be was in Oldham a month or so later while she was at the clinic in Oldham. She had just finished having a crafty cigarette by the window and went back to her bed and picked up a puzzle book. Mr. Steptoe came in to see her and said: "Have you seen the papers today?" Mum replied "No" and he said: "There are some stories going round in the papers. At the moment they are just talking about a woman in Oldham.

I'm not happy for you to be here in case the press find you. I want to send you home so can you get in contact with John."

Patrick Steptoe said he would take Mum to the station if she could arrange for Dad to meet her at Temple Meads in Bristol. Mr. Steptoe and his wife took her to the station and put her on the train. The fact that a doctor seemed so worried that she might be spotted by the press and escorted her personally to the station with his wife brought home to her the fact that this was no ordinary pregnancy.

When she got to Temple Meads she walked with her suitcase towards Newtown near Trinity Road Police station in Bristol. Halfway there she stopped at the Rediffusion television rental shop where her sister-in-law worked and was able to leave the case there before walking the rest of the way home. Patrick Steptoe and Bob Edwards would have gone crazy if they had known - Dad certainly did when he saw his hot and bothered wife arrive home unexpectedly after a train journey and long walk!

In the last three months of Mum's pregnancy the media fuss got bigger and bigger.

As speculation grew and bits and pieces of information about the event began to be pieced together by the media Mum was booked into Oldham General Hospital under the name Rita Ferguson and staff there given a false address in Oldham for her by Steptoe. Few of them knew that she had become pregnant through IVF and that my conception had taken place in a laboratory overseen by Edwards.

Just a small number of senior staff knew that "Rita" was in fact the "test-tube baby mum" that the constant stream of journalists besieging the hospital were trying to find. The "Fergusons" also booked into some nearby guest-houses at times and some of Mum's relatives were in on the code-name - sending her letters in that name and talking about her on the phone as Rita!

In the few weeks before I was born the story had gone global and reporters from America and Japan had flown to the UK and joined the national media in trying to find out as much as they could about this

British woman that was going to have a baby in such a sensational way. There had never been a baby conceived in the history of the world in this way. It was a medical science breakthrough but also threw up lots of religious and moral questions in different cultures around the world.

In those weeks Mum saw little of the newspaper coverage as she was hidden away in the hospital. She really only realised the fuss that was going on outside when she received flowers out of the blue at her hospital ward from the Daily Express. Of course they were just trying to get friendly to get the story.

Patrick Steptoe had used a well-established firm of lawyers in Oldham called Wrigley Claydon and Armstrong, who were based in Prudential Buildings in Union Street. Patrick took Dad along to meet Paul Vincent, who was one of their partners. Paul had previously drawn up various legal agreements to do with Steptoe's IVF work.

Mum and Dad had little experience of legal affairs and Paul Vincent became their lawyer and he was tasked with the job of trying to do some kind of deal with the media. There were offers and counter-offers being made and a frenzy of media interest surrounded the hospital.

Paul Vincent himself became a target of media interest with press people camped out in the reception area of Prudential Buildings, surrounding him and asking him for the latest news of Mum and Dad.

Under pressure and to try to protect Mum, the men: Dad, Bob Edwards, Patrick Steptoe and Paul Vincent agreed to do a deal with the Daily Mail giving them an exclusive on the birth. In return the newspaper promised to protect Mum and Dad from the media scrum, which of course would also protect their world exclusive story if and when I was born. The Daily Mail also found Dad a place to stay - up until then he had often slept in the car to save money or in a cheap bed and breakfast when he had some money. The Daily Mail sent reporters to stay with Dad, so say to look after him but really to ensure that their story was protected and he didn't speak to anyone else.

The Daily Mail were so keen to keep their exclusive that they took to smuggling Dad into Paul Vincent's office under a blanket. In fact there was so much fuss around the office that much of the legal agreement was done at Paul Vincent's home in nearby Waterhead. The main agreement with the Daily Mail was signed at 2.30am in his kitchen.

So much was reported about how much that deal was worth but most of those reports were greatly exaggerated. Mum and Dad had spent so much of their lives close to the breadline that any deal giving them money was likely to be attractive, especially if it meant they could afford to buy the baby equipment they needed. They were also fearful of facing the media alone - and the Daily Mail offered them protection. News of the exclusive only fueled the media speculation and antics of the reporters.

The most embarrassing and disgusting moment was when a desperate journalist trying to get the story rang the hospital saying there was a bomb in the building. Patients were evacuated, operations were stopped. That journalist could have killed someone and shows the stupid lengths that journalists would go to in order to get their story. Mum was wheeled out anonymously and not spotted.

As the days went on expectation grew about the birth. The newspapers got more and more excited. The Daily Mail brought Mum's Mum and her partner to the hospital for a visit. Members of staff at the hospital, including nurses were being offered money in local pubs to tell stories about the "test-tube baby mum". The fact the Daily Mail had an exclusive deal just angered the other national newspapers who became increasingly desperate to wreck the story and find their own angle on it. Mum was blissfully unaware of all this as by now she had been put into a room on her own. Papers weren't allowed in and everything sent into her was being censored and checked. Dad was drinking and chatting with the journalists from the Daily Mail, who were being friendly to him but all the time getting more and more bits of information to put into their story. With Mum and Dad's background it was easy to impress them with a nice meal or item of clothing for Mum. All peanuts to the big international newspaper group, who knew just how valuable the story would be to them worldwide.

In the days just before my birth Mum got bored sitting in the little room in isolation, only going out to other parts of the hospital for tests. She had her own bathroom and Dad brought a small television from home.

Nets were put up to the window to stop photographers taking pictures of her in her room from nearby buildings.

July 25 came and Mum had gone for a scan and Patrick Steptoe came into the room and said: "Lesley, I think it is about time the baby was born." He told Mum not to tell anyone, not even Dad or the nursing staff. He said he would telephone Dad and let him know about the plans.

Because Dad was staying with the Daily Mail reporters it was feared that they would try to get into the hospital if they knew the cesarean section was about to take place. Patrick Steptoe only told his closest confidantes about the plans for the day. There was a real fear that if any member of staff knew they might tell one of the media organisations just to get some money.

As Mum was about to have a cesarean section she wasn't allowed to eat but Patrick Steptoe could not put the usual sign up saying "Nil by mouth" as that would have given away the plans to the nurses and other staff.

Lunch was duly delivered and Patrick Steptoe arranged for his wife Sheena to visit Mum. The two of them giggled as they poured the lunchtime drinks down the sink and Sheena put the food into bags she had smuggled in and took them away in her handbag.

Dad and Sharon came in for a visit in the afternoon and Mum just couldn't keep it a secret from them. She told him that the baby was going to be born that night but swore them to secrecy and at the end of the visit they were whisked off with their Daily Mail minders to a flat nearby where the newspaper was keeping them so that other media couldn't get near them.

Later the theatre sister Edith Astell came into the room. She turned the lights off so that all staff in the area thought that Mum had been settled down for the night. She took out a torch and prepared Mum for the operation by torchlight. The two women giggled at the conspiracy going on. Edith Astell even attached a catheter to Mum ready for the operation by the light of her torch. They whispered and laughed and then Edith left and told Mum to pretend to be asleep if anyone came in.

Mum lay in the dark and soon she was collected to be taken to the operating theatre. As she was wheeled through the corridors all along the route she saw rows and rows of police officers all along the route from her room to the theatre.

The anaesthetic was delivered and the next thing Mum knew was someone saying: "Lesley, do you want to see your baby? It's a little girl." She saw a fuzzy outline of me and fell asleep again until the next day.

I had been born. The medical team called me "normal" but that wasn't the way the press wanted to portray it. Within hours headlines were around the world declaring that a "miracle baby" had been born.

Chapter 3

WORLD REACTION

I got my first proposal of marriage when I was just five days old lying in my cot in the maternity unit at Oldham Hospital. It came in the form of a blue air-mail letter addressed to my Mum C/O Dr. Patrick Steptoe, Oldham General Hospital (Maternity Ward) and was from New Delhi.

The sender was a 21-year-old chap called Harry Bansi. It might seem a bit strange but in a way the letter was quite sweet.

It read: "Hiya. Here's wishing you most hearty congratulations on the birth of your baby girl. It has been a great achievement for science and a personal triumph for you. I hope and pray that your baby may live a normal and healthy life. And even though I'm already 21 years old, I'd still like to have the privilege of being the first man to propose marriage to her. If she may want me when she grows up."

I never did look up Harry later in life but it is nice to be wanted! The letter does show what a huge impact the story was having on the world and it was one of more than 400 letters, cards and telegrams that Mum received while in Oldham Hospital for 12 long days following my birth.

Most people when they have their first baby can find things get a bit tiring with so many relatives wanting to pop in and see the little one. Aunts and uncles, cousins and friends all want to see the baby and have a cuddle.

It can all get a little too much and a bit exhausting at times when all you want is to be alone with your baby and get used to feeding it, changing its nappy and just staring at how perfect it is!

It's especially hard for first-time mums as there is nothing quite so terrifying as finding yourself in charge of a precious little human life for the first time. So imagine what it was like for my Mum with the world's media writing about her and Dad. The hospital was under siege from the media and decisions needed to be made about what to do about this "miracle" baby that was causing so much excitement.

My birth had prompted debates about all sorts of things. Some people were arguing about whether it was against God and religion to bring a baby into the world this way; some people were discussing the rights and wrongs of "cheque-book journalism" saying that it was wrong for one media organisation to have control of such an important story; some people were excited by the scientific and medical breakthrough; some believed it was the start of cloning or designer babies. Mum and Dad just wanted to be left alone with their older daughter Sharon and the new baby - the baby they had been trying for for years.

The discussions and debates were going on all over the world. The day before I was born Time Magazine in New York published an article about my birth saying: "Some are sure to see in the world's first test-tube infant visions of the baby hatcheries in Aldous Huxley's Brave New World. The expected birth has already become a press circus."

The next week's edition saw my birth as the cover story in Time magazine with the headline "The Test-tube Baby" and "Birth watch in Britain" and no less than eight pages dedicated to the story inside. The description from their reporter gives some idea of what it must have been like to be in that hospital:

"Normally quiet Oldham (pop 227,000) last week was in a state of siege. From as far off as Japan, scores of reporters and cameramen had converged on the town to be on hand for the birth of Baby Brown.

Despite pleas from the doctors that the hulabaloo was endangering both mother and child, journalists steadfastly prowled the hospital's precincts. They were seeking any morsel of news. Perhaps a brief word with one of the doctors responsible for the Brown's experiment; Patrick Steptoe who came and went daily in his white Mercedes, dodging in and out of the hospital's side doors to avoid the press. Or a chat with the equally elusive Father. Or, scoop of scoops, a photograph of Lesley Brown peeking from behind her carefully curtained window."

Other pages looked at the ethics of the birth; a cartoon showing two children playing with a chemistry set with the caption: "They're playing mother's and fathers" illustrated one page and there was a whole page dedicated to the "frenzy" going on in the British press. It was that frenzy that was causing Mum and Dad the most problems.

Just a week or so before I was born Dad would often go to the local pub in Oldham and would sit a few feet from many of the reporters who were looking for him. Few had any idea what he looked like until his picture was splashed over the papers a few days before I was born.

Of course the first thing the press wanted to know was the name of the new baby. Short of a story the papers had speculated that I would be called Patricia in honour of Patrick Steptoe or Roberta after Robert Edwards. Mum didn't like either name. Nobody is quite sure where Louise came from but that was what I was called. It was Patrick Steptoe that suggested "Joy" as a middle name as he said my birth would bring so much joy to the world as it gave hope for childless couples everywhere.

In America it was widely reported that I was called Patricia - to such an extent that many of the telegrams, cards and letters from well-wishers in America talked about "baby Patricia" or wishing Mum well in bringing up Roberta!

My birth seemed to bring out the worst in all the journalists. This was hardly a story that needed sensationalising. Nobody had ever been born this way and the work of Patrick Steptoe and Robert Edwards should have been celebrated by the media for what it was - one of the great medical breakthroughs in history.

Instead what was reported was a lot of wrangles and pathetic one-upmanship by the newspapers. The rivalry between the Daily Express and the Daily Mail got very heated.

Derek Jameson, legendary editor of the Daily Express was particularly angry that a deal had been done with the Daily Mail. He was quoted as saying: "This story is bigger than man conquering the moon. For the Mail to insist they had the exclusive - that's like buying up Louis Pasteur and then saying you can only buy antiseptics through the Daily Mail syndication department."

Frustrated at not being the first people to have the full story he hit out at Mum and Dad and the doctors saying daft things like: "We could get baby farms, mass produced kids, 1984 six years early."

I don't expect he meant it and as far as the editors were concerned it was all banter aimed at getting one over on a rival publication. But the number of thoughtless comments by journalists trying to fill column inches with speculation and ill-informed debate had an effect on people all over the world, who then turned on Mum and Dad and the doctors and started sending hate mail and saying awful things about them.

The media excitement has followed me all of my life. It is only in recent years that people have started to question the methods and morals of the press. Certainly in 1978 tabloid journalism was at its height; cheque-book journalism - where people bought stories for money - was in full flow. The National Enquirer in the USA were said to have sent six reporters half way round the world to try to buy up the story.

The real media battle between the Mail and the Express had kicked off two weeks before I was born.

Someone at the Express must have found out that the Daily Mail were close to Steptoe and Edwards so on July 11 they ran a front page story with the headline: "Baby Of The Century".

It called Mum "Mrs A" and said pompously: "The Daily Express knows the woman's identity but has not named her at this stage for ethical reasons." More important in the story they published was the fact that the British Medical Association Central Ethical Committee had approved of the IVF process as a new form of treatment for infertile women.

The rest of the "Express World Exclusive" was what most journalists would call "a spoiler". Bits of tittle-tattle gleaned from knocking on the doors of neighbours of Mum and Dad and chatting to a few of Dad's workmates were dressed up as quotes from Mum and Dad. The main aim was to make it look like they had the full story and so devalue the Mail "exclusive".

Patrick Steptoe was clearly out of his depth in handling the media and a statement was written for him by the Daily Mail that said: "Myself, my colleagues and the medical and nursing team involved in the forthcoming birth at Oldham wish to state that pressure by the media could endanger our patient and her child. This makes this morning's lapse by one newspaper even more regrettable. I happen to know that many of its rivals could have published all that they printed and more but exercised restraint with the well-being of our patient in mind."

The Daily Mail and Associated Newspapers fanned the flames of outrage by saying all information would be issued through them first. This just made every other journalist publish any old piece of rubbish they could find.

There were enough clues in the Express story to make the Daily Mail feel that they knew Mum and Dad so the next day the Mail published the names of Mum and Dad and the gloves were off. Amazingly The Sun also published the names the same day - showing that the journalists were all closing in on the story at the same time.

With Mum and Dad named in two of its rivals the Express decided that its "ethical" reasons were no longer valid. They published a picture of Dad secretly snatched in the hospital car park. They quoted him saying a few sentences, like "God I wish it were all over" and "All we want is to be a normal family." I suspect they were things he said to reporters who collared him in a pub the night before to try to get rid of them. The fact they hadn't spoken to Dad was clear by the fact that they called him Gilbert - his real first name but one he would never use and one he would never say was his name, if asked!

Things were getting silly with journalists making up amounts that they believed the exclusive deal with the Daily Mail was worth, politicians then commenting on those figures as if they were fact and even saying that it wasn't right that money should be changing hands while Mum and Dad were getting NHS treatment.

In fact Mum and Dad had to pay for a lot of the early treatment and really only got NHS care around the birth - which was the same as anyone else having a baby would get. Then because of the newspaper fuss Mum had been moved into a private ward and had to pay bills for every night of special accommodation that she got.

The newspaper fees did help them financially but when you realise how much they had to pay out to get this baby through the private treatment, how much time they lost at work unpaid because they were unable to get to work because of the journalists there and then all the extra costs of things like security and transport because of the world-wide interest it wasn't exactly something they would have been able to finance without the media deal.

So what exactly was that media deal that caused all the fuss? At no time in my life did Mum and Dad tell me anything about the deal. I never received any money as I grew up from that media deal. I can only go by the documents that my parents had - originals drawn up by the lawyer Paul Vincent and signed by all parties.

It was widely reported that my parents received £325,000 for the exclusive rights to their story. I believe that figure was made up by the Daily Express and then repeated in newspapers throughout Britain and the USA until people just repeated it as if it was true. The Daily Mirror were so obsessed by the amounts they believed the family were getting for the story of my birth that when I was born they spelt my name Louise with a £ for the first letter - £ouise!

In fact the original agreement was signed as late as July 14th - just two weeks before I was born and when the press had already been saying for three months that a mega-deal had been signed. On that day Mum and Dad were persuaded by the lawyers to become directors of a company called Chandlewise and that from the company they would each get £250 a month salary for the next seven years plus a car.

It was explained to them that this would help them with tax issues and would enable money to be paid to the company for any films, books and other offers. The company could then pay for any expenses incurred. It meant Mum and Dad would get £6,000 a year between them - the average UK salary in 1978 was £5,500 so it wasn't megabucks by anyone's standards. Of course Dad was also keen to keep his job on the railway and the car would come in handy so they saw it as a good deal.

With the company in place money could be paid to it as and when offers came in. Any expenses that came about as a result of all the fuss - such as transport or security - could be paid for by the company. Steptoe, Edwards and Paul Vincent had been persuaded by the media fuss that there could be income in the future from advertising endorsements, film rights and books about the birth.

Associated Newspapers Group agreed to pay £6,000 to the company straight away on July 14 and another £4,000 provided the baby was born alive. As long as Mum and Dad didn't allow themselves to be photographed or give any interviews to anyone else and as long as the baby was not "significantly malformed or mentally retarded and is generally healthy and normal" and provided Mum and Dad had allowed the newspaper to publish their exclusive story within five days of the birth then a further £20,000 would be paid two weeks after my birth.

Another £15,000 would be paid when Mum left hospital provided the newspaper had that event as an exclusive and a further £15,000 would be paid another 28 days later providing Mum and Dad did not do interviews or photographs with others.

That means that Associated Newspapers agreed to pay a total of £60,000 to the company - enough to pay Mum and Dad for the next 10 years on the deal they had - within a month or so of my birth.

It was impressed upon Mum and Dad that the money would only be forthcoming if they could avoid the many reporters that were besieging the hospital, their home, their family members and popping up just about everywhere. Although it was more money than they had ever had in their lives, far from taking the pressure off Mum and Dad it actually made things worse for them and just made the media even more keen to find them and write about them.

The week before I was born the Oldham Area Health Authority Administrator was reported as saying that Mum might be moved out of the hospital because of the media pressure.

He told reporter David Thomas: "The number of press reporters at the hospital is making the situation extremely difficult for us. It seems if you move anything there is a reporter behind it. One reporter had the nerve to pose as a visitor and go in wards questioning patients. That sort of thing is intolerable."

This only prompted reporters to set up camp at St Mary's Hospital, Manchester and Highfield Private Nursing Home in Rochdale - both places where they were speculating that I might be born if it was decided to move Mum away from Oldham.

There is no doubt looking back that the media situation wasn't handled well. On July 13 the Daily Express published a blurry photograph of Mum that was years old under the banner headline: "The Test-tube Mum".

Journalist Harry Pugh gushed: "Here she is - the woman the world has been waiting to see." They had stopped calling Dad Gilbert though and were calling him John. The rest of the story was mostly MPs criticising the "£325,000" deal with the Daily Mail. Remember, at that time no deal had been signed with anyone! It wasn't signed until the day after!

Among Mum's favourite cuttings is one labelled "Another Sun

Exclusive" and written by Charles Garside - the journalist who really was the first to track down Mum and Dad to their home but missed out after that. The headline reads: "Test-tube Baby Boy" and with the sub-heading saying: "It's a lad forecast as hospital makes a scan check."

The story is based on the fact that staff at the hospital were heard referring to the baby as "he" after a scan check on Mum. It says the boy will be born in the first week of August and will be christened Patrick after Patrick Steptoe.

The story goes on to say that Mum and Dad were planning to move into a new home financed by the £325,000 they are about to receive and that they are also about to get "fabulous offers from advertisement agencies, television producers and authors."

The press did everything to put pressure on the Daily Mail. In the days leading up to my birth Dad had a couple of Daily Mail minders living with him in a flat nearby and Mum also had some protection allocated to her to prevent journalists getting to her. Other media organisations engineered complaints about the Daily Mail "guards" on Mum's room so they were replaced by hospital security staff. Then they prompted rows about the costs of those security men.

Then Paul Vincent got involved in a row over the film. The day after I was born pressure was put on the Government to release the film to the TV channels as it had been taken by the Central Office of Information, which as part of the Government is funded by the taxpayer. Paul Vincent said the last minute deal had expressly said that the film couldn't be shown for 28 days (to protect the Mail's exclusive). He took out an injunction on behalf of the Daily Mail against the Government and it was only after he had a telephone conversation with the Minister of Health Roland Moyle that the Government backed down.

Amidst all of this Dad was reeling from the fact that he had a new baby. He was reported by many newspapers as "mumbling incoherently" or "blubbing". Sharon went to buy a three foot teddy bear for her sister, which my son Cameron has to this day. It featured in newspapers all around the world.

Mum had to recover from the full anaesthetic and get used to looking after a baby so she was also kept out of the spotlight for those first few days. Dad did a press conference which was attended by all media to try to take the media pressure off but with no appearance from Mum or me the press frenzy continued.

The fuss all over the world had certainly made the pound signs jump up and down in the corridors of power at Associated Newspapers, publishers of the Daily Mail. The original contract they had negotiated with Paul Vincent had been signed by Dad on July 14 - some 10 days before I was born.

At that time Dad had agreed that he and Mum wouldn't talk to any other media without the Daily Mail's permission for 28 days after Mum left hospital, but while Mum was still recovering at the hospital from having me they had realised that the story had a lot more interest than even they had originally thought. The Daily Mail lawyers set to drawing up another contract and negotiating once again with Paul Vincent.

This contract tied Mum and Dad to Associated Newspapers for 400 days after my birth and was signed by Mum. They were keen to make sure that they were the people who had the "exclusive" story when I was one year old - so had timed the contract to take the story past my first birthday. Having sold on the rights to the birth to the National Enquirer they could see this being a source of income for the next year.

Associated Newspapers also wanted to make sure that any other milestones during my first year of life were reported first in their newspapers - so the agreement was that Mum and Dad would co-operate with up to five interviews, the last one being around my first birthday. The company Chandlewise would get £500 for each interview over the course of the next year.

The contract in its legal jargon also said no photographs were allowed to be taken of me or Mum and Dad without the permission of Associated Newspapers. The contract effectively meant that even if a member of our family took a picture of Mum or Dad the newspaper had to be informed and give their consent. If they weren't then the paper was entitled to keep its £500 payments for the interviews.

The five page typed document was called a "supplemental agreement" and I don't think in reality Mum had much idea what it was all about. The only bits she really took in were the fact that they might get some money, the fact that she wasn't allowed to talk to the media and the fact that the lawyers and media people promised to look after her with all the fuss going on.

Unlike today's multi-media world where everyone is online as well as in print Associated Newspapers were only really interested in the newspaper world. The contract allowed Mum and Dad to co-operate with others for a book, to get involved in any advertising and in any films or television programmes (as long as Associated Newspapers had approved of the projects first of course). Of course Mum and Dad were just continuing to receive the £250 a month each from Chandlewise.

After a few days Mum just wanted to get home and get back to some kind of normality. The Daily Mail brought relatives to see her but they were more worried about getting photos to keep the story going in the newspaper than her welfare. Patrick Steptoe was pleased that the deal with the newspaper had at least kept the full force of the media away from Mum but really it was all out of control.

Back in Bristol relatives were being collared by journalists and just about every religious leader, politician or medical expert was being telephoned and questioned about their view of the "test-tube baby". Each statement being rolled out as another "exclusive". In reality all that was happening was that Mum was slowly recovering, I was snuggled in a cot like every other baby and the hospital was just trying to behave as if nothing unusual had happened.

In her little room Mum was away from most of the fuss. She put on her frilly nightie and washed her hair and held me for photographs for the Daily Mail. They had sold the North American rights to the story to the National Enquirer, probably turning a swift profit on their "exclusive".

The American newspaper reporter and photographer arrived at the hospital ward armed with a cardboard sign printed with the words: "Congratulations to the most special baby in the world from readers of the National Enquirer" which they propped up behind Mum as she cradled me in her arms. This was to ensure others couldn't copy the photograph without advertising their newspaper - you have to remember this was a long time before Photoshop and digital pictures!

The report they produced in the National Enquirer was the only one that upset Mum. It was a bit that read: "Within hours of her birth, Louise proved herself a perfect nuisance - crying so loudly that she woke up all the other infants in her nursery and they started screaming too. Nurses promptly nicknamed her "Big Mouth".

"She's got lungs like a glassblower", said one nurse. "She's bound to become a pop singer or politician!"

Mum was tearful at her precious bundle being called "Big Mouth". I must admit I have been called worse since then and maybe Mum was just suffering from a bit of post-natal tearfulness or the effects of the anaesthetic - whatever it was she remembered it as the worst moment in dealing with the press in those days in hospital.

She was shocked to see cuttings arrive at the ward from newspapers in Bombay and Dunedin in New Zealand and even cuttings in Japanese. She pasted them all in a big scrapbook.

Telegrams were arriving daily from neighbours in Hassell Drive, Bristol, from friends and relatives, from Charles Garside at The Sun, from complete strangers and from famous people like the pop group Herman's Hermits. They wrote: "Mrs Brown You've got a lovely daughter congratulations stop we did it 12 years ago but ours went round and round and played at 45rpm stop all the best from Herman's Hermits." They were referring, of course, to the title of their own hit record.

Mum was surprised to get a telegram from the Bristol MP Arthur

Palmer. The cards were now filling up the little room in the hospital. Mum barely had time to look at them all - some had messages from relatives and friends, some had come from the other side of the world. It was scary.

The nurses started putting the cards on a little bedside table, then sticking them to the door and as the days went on the walls of the little room were entirely covered with cards and greetings from all corners of the globe.

But the worldwide interest in the birth meant it wasn't going to be easy to get home and Mum was getting bored in hospital. She was crying a lot of the time now on a couple of occasions telling Dad that she just wanted to go home. With all the fuss it was hard for them to just live normally. After 12 long days it was decided to move us home to Bristol - the medics had done all their tests on me and Mum was fully recovered. Mum knew the journey would be a bit of an ordeal and had been warned about the media - deep down though she was more worried about looking after a baby on her own for the first time without the hospital staff around her - the fears that every mum has when baby is new.

Dad was taken to Kershaw's Cottage Hospital in Oldham where he thanked everyone for the work they had done in making Mum pregnant. Mum said her goodbyes to Patrick Steptoe and she said he was very emotional telling her to "look after me" because I was "special".

Gifts including the giant teddy bear and a huge costume doll that had been sent by the Brazilian Embassy on behalf of that country and a magnificent ornate wooden cot that had arrived "from the people of Turkey" all had to be packed up to be taken the 180 miles to Bristol. There had been a constant media presence outside the hospital since my birth and word soon got around that I was finally going home and might put in an appearance in the outside world. An ambulance was pulled up outside the hospital and it was soon surrounded by photographers, TV crews and reporters. I was carried into the big wide world for the first time in my Mum's arms, wrapped in a shawl. Flashbulbs went off and questions were shouted from a mob of journalists as Mum, surrounded by hospital staff, carried her baby to the ambulance. Lawyer Paul Vincent was there along with minders from the Daily Mail preventing reporters from getting too close to Mum and me.

Once inside the ambulance was surrounded by the mob of journalists holding cameras up to the windows and taking flash pictures at random. A Daily Mail reporter climbed into the back of the ambulance - they were determined that other newspapers and news media wouldn't get a decent photograph of me at that stage.

The ambulance driver pulled down blinds on the windows to stop the photographers getting a view. Mum was more worried about the bright flashbulbs damaging her new born baby's eyes.

On the journey back to Bristol the ambulance stopped at a motorway services as Mum was dying for a cup of tea. The Daily Mail reporter wouldn't let Mum go into the cafe in case she was recognised. I was left in the care of the ambulance driver while Mum and the man from the Daily Mail had a cup of tea in an area reserved for the police!

Word came over the ambulance radio that our house in Hassell Drive was under siege from the media so the driver pulled in to a deserted speedway track on the outskirts of Bristol in the hope that things might calm down.

While the world's press were waiting outside Mum's house I was blissfully having a feed just a few miles down the road before dozing off into a nice sleep. But it was all very frustrating for Mum, so near to getting home but told to wait there while the police and people from the Daily Mail tried to work out how to get her into her own house with her new baby.

Eventually the ambulance driver and Mum decided to make a dash for it. Sure enough there was a huge crowd of people outside the house - not only the media but neighbours and others who had heard the "test-tube baby" was coming home and just wanted to be part of this big news event.

The ambulance driver lifted me in a carry-cot above everyone's heads and carried me into the house. Mum tried to put her cardigan on but it got caught over her head as television cameras and a microphone on a long pole were pushed into the ambulance as soon as the doors opened. It was chaos. Some reports said Mum was hiding her face as she left the ambulance but it was simply the fact that she was being bundled around and unable to put her cardigan on properly!

BBC television reporter Malcolm Frith tried to get close to the ambulance with his cameraman and had his arm slammed in the door by the Daily Mail minders that were on duty. He screamed in pain but couldn't be heard above the noise so had to punch the man responsible for trapping him and that started a scuffle. It was scary for Mum and frightening for Dad, who was worried about my safety in it all.

Finally with some pushing and pulling Mum made it to the house too. But inside was hardly an oasis of clam. As well as the immediate family there were Daily Mail reporters, minders and a photographer capturing the special moment. It was no way for a Mum to return home with her newborn baby.

The reporters from other papers were besicging the house, standing in the garden, pressing their faces up against the windows and taking photos through them so the Daily Mail - who were now more like bodyguards than reporters - dragged everyone upstairs.

So there was Mum home for the first time with her new baby. No time to put the kettle on or see close family as the Daily Mail wanted to do a photoshoot of me in my nursery cot for the first time, while outside all hell was breaking loose with people pushing and shoving, the road blocked, police being called to control the crowds and photographers paying people in the houses opposite so they could train their lenses on the bedroom windows in an attempt to ruin the Daily Mail's "exclusive".

Mum and Dad apparently had a bit of a row because Dad had forgotten to put a net curtain back up in my bedroom after painting it so that had to be hastily put back to keep the prying eyes out. Sharon was caught up in all the confusion and was photographed glaring out of the window at the lunatic antics of the world's media.

Of course Mum and Dad never really knew what media was outside the house but I have heard that people travelled from all over the world to stand outside that little house in Hassell Drive and not get any pictures of me or any words from Mum or Dad. They filled the gap with gossip from neighbours and anyone else with an opinion about whether having a "test-tube baby" was a good or a bad thing.

There were stories that some people made money out of giving bits and pieces of information about my family to the press. Certainly some made a few bob out of letting photographers use their bedrooms to get a view of the street. Good luck to them but it showed the idiocy of the media frenzy around my birth. Little did we know that this was just the beginning of the media circus that was to follow me all my life.

Chapter 4

UNDER SIEGE IN HASSELL DRIVE!

A s a teenager with a new baby sister Sharon was in her element. She loved helping Mum look after the new baby and with so much fuss going on around the family she became very protective of me. Mum was grateful of the help most of the time, although I know they had a few clashes with Sharon wanting to help out and Mum keen to look after her own baby.

Although the Daily Mail had now published its exclusive and the whole world knew about me, the newspaper was determined to milk its agreement to the maximum. Told that they could lose out on thousands of pounds if they let themselves be interviewed or photographed Mum and Dad were virtual prisoners in their own home. For the first few weeks a guard from the Daily Mail answered the door to all callers, who were mostly reporters from other publications and the postman bringing sacks full of mail from all around the world.

The newspaper had done a deal with Stern magazine in Germany, which had a big close-up of me on the cover on August 4 and Australian Woman's Weekly published an "exclusive" on August 16 with a picture of me Mum and Dad taken in hospital in Oldham on the cover.

Inside the pages of articles included an interview with Mum's Mum...

my Nanny Jean by the renowned journalist Lynda Lee-Potter about why she had left Mum as a baby. It seems my birth had brought them close together once more and Nanny Jean became a really important part of my childhood. There wasn't a corner of the world where Mum's story and my picture wasn't being syndicated by the newspaper.

That didn't mean that the media left Mum alone. They set up camp in Hassell Drive, knocking on the door all the time to ask for photographs, comments or some information. Basically Mum and Dad had said everything there was to say but every newspaper, magazine and TV station somehow had their own daft question that they wanted to ask.

The American television network CBS had its first female correspondent Susan Peterson in London and she was duly dispatched to Bristol. I guess they felt that a woman's touch might help with this particular story. But she found herself joining the mob sitting outside Hassell Drive looking at the drawn curtains and occasionally getting excited when Dad left to visit someone or a relative arrived or someone authorised by the Daily Mail got let in through the front door.

The day after I arrived home she pushed a note through the door. Frustrated at the fact that Mum hadn't shown her face she had a cunning plan.

The note read: "If you don't want to do an interview - for whatever reasons - I completely understand... but if you could give us a definite answer one way or another, it would be helpful.

"You see if we have a definite refusal it helps us convince our editors to give up - and leave you and your family in peace. (A nod - up or down - out the window would be enough - if you don't want to open the door!)"

The television and stills cameras were then trained on the window hoping that Mum would be daft enough to stick her head out of the window and shake it from side to side. You have to laugh!

After a few days Susan Peterson had appointed herself leader of a little coalition of television journalists. Joined by Graham Purches the local BBC reporter, Simon Bucks of HTV West and Ken Rees of ITN they wrote another note.

It read: "I have talked to all the reporters outside and all have agreed to leave if you could only say a few words to us (outside or inside) about the baby and how she's doing - or at least allow us a brief picture of the baby.

"We stress that the last thing any of us want to do is to cause any unnecessary aggravation to yourselves and the rest of the family. If granted, our request would only take a few minutes - and then we could leave you in peace."

The siege continued despite the fact that just about every detail of the story had now been published in every country imaginable. It became a crazy game of cat and mouse between the family and the press - Sharon of course was more protective than anyone else and became expert at spotting journalists and their wheedling tactics.

Of course the press siege was not just fuelled by curiosity to see this new baby. My birth had caused a worldwide sensation and thrown up all kinds of moral and religious arguments. Mum and Dad were basically Christian. Like most British people in those days they had been brought up learning all about God and Jesus but they didn't go to church regularly and they had no particularly strongly held beliefs other than to try to treat people decently and do the right thing.

Moral issues had never been discussed when they were thinking of having a baby. They were old-fashioned in the fact that they didn't want to have a baby "out of wedlock" so they had waited until they were married to try for a baby. They had never once discussed whether what Patrick Steptoe and Robert Edwards were doing was morally right or wrong. All they were interested in was having a baby and if these medical people could come up with a way to help Mum do that they were happy to take part in the IVF programme.

But in areas of the world with strong religious faith I was a real threat. Only one person - Jesus Christ - had ever claimed to be born without a couple having sex and he was the Son of God. Some religions believed that if a woman or a man couldn't have a baby then that was "God's will" and by finding a way around that then the doctors were "playing God" and messing with the natural order of things.

Many people believed that I couldn't possibly be normal and as the doctors had checked out that I was physically the same as everyone else they decided there must be something else wrong with me. Some decided that I would develop abnormally and die young or have some awful illness. Others decided I must be possessed of some super-powers or on the other hand have some behavioural problems, of course none of it was true. I was just a normal healthy baby. The fact I was hidden away by the papers added to the mystery and led to more speculation. Some religious groups decided that the thing I would be lacking would be a soul - they said that vital bit of a human being couldn't possibly be added in a test-tube or petri dish.

One group of fanatics in the USA said that on the day I was born the Virgin Mary appeared and gave them a message saying: "It is an abomination in the eyes of God for man in his arrogance and pride to seek to create the living being. What he is creating is a soulless monster, a being of destruction for all that it will meet. I say "it", for it is not truly a human being but 'a thing', my children, a thing!"

The full wrath of the religious leaders was really aimed at Edwards and Steptoe. Thirty years before the Nazis had wanted to create perfect babies for Hitler's Europe and had carried out experiments in concentration camps in Poland and elsewhere - the work of Steptoe and Edwards was being unfairly aligned with these awful events.

The combination of the protectiveness of the Daily Mail and Mum's natural shyness and fear of the spotlight meant speculation grew. Here is one report that was printed in America at the time and which is still doing the rounds on the internet:

Six weeks old, the miracle Test-tube Baby of England can move solid objects with its mind and shows it can read the thoughts of others.

These are the amazing reports coming from Bristol, England, where baby Louise Brown now lives under heavy guard with her parents, Gilbert and Lesley Brown.

The infant, born July 25, began showing alarming psychic abilities shortly after coming home from Oldham General Hospital.

'Baby Louise looked at a teddy bear on a shelf near her crib. The doll slid off, onto the floor,' confided George Landingham, one of the security hired by the London Daily Mail to protect the Brown home. The Daily Mail has exclusive rights to all stories and photos about the world's first test-tube baby.

'The same day, the mother carried a stack of clean diapers into the nursery. She was holding them firmly at the top and bottom of the stack. But suddenly they slid out of her hands.

'Mrs. Brown said she felt an unseen force tug the diapers out of her hand. Then she noticed baby Louise was staring oddly in her direction.'

The guard said Mrs. Brown went into near panic when she entered the nursery first thing one morning, and found all the furniture pulled away from the walls.

'A chest of drawers was in the middle of the room, 10 feet from its normal position,' he reveals. 'A nightstand which had been near the crib was on the other side of the room, completely turned around. A picture on the wall had fallen to the floor.

'Yet no one had been in the room for the past six hours, when the baby had its 2 a.m. feeding.'

In the first few days after baby Louise came home, the only visitors besides relatives were medical representatives of Oldham Hospital, making regular medical checks on the infant's progress.

They included Dr. James Durrville-Smith chief of neurosurgery at London College of Medicine; Dr. Winston P. Nicolson, chief of psychiatry at the same institution; Dr. Laurence Attenborough, brain specialist from Liverpool; and Dr. Manfred J. Lichtenstein, German-born psychiatrist generally considered to be Britain's top expert in paranormal brain activity.

All except Dr. Lichtenstein have refused comment on the nature of their visits to the Brown home. He stated carefully: 'Problems concerning *the baby's mental development have arisen. Certain things have occurred which were totally unforeseen.'*

'Physically, the baby is healthy and normal. The problem involves what appears to be a highly irregular brain abnormality.' Asked if the Brown infant were retarded, the doctor snapped: 'Quite the opposite!' He refused to answer more questions.

The same group of doctors, plus others, has been seen entering the offices of Dr. Patrick Steptoe, the famed gynaecologist who performed the breakthrough procedure of fertilizing an ovum from Mrs. Brown outside her body.

Dr. Steptoe and his colleague, Dr. Edwards, are completely incognito since rumors of strange mental powers in the Brown baby began to be heard.

The guard detail around the Brown's modest home in a working class neighborhood of Bristol has been doubled. Even the IDs of close relatives are constantly checked and rechecked.

'All I know is that it's easier to get into the Queen's private chambers at Buckingham Palace than into the Brown's front yard,' groused Charlie Parham, who lives next door.

'You hear the strangest stories. I heard one of the security men say that the baby appears to be able to read her mum's mind. For instance, when Mrs. Brown thinks that it's time for the baby's feeding, the baby stops fretting even before she moves toward the kitchen.'

In London, Dr. Fredric Sykes, a genetics expert who long has opposed the procedure which brought Mrs. Brown a baby daughter, said that the parents and Dr. Steptoe deserve the consequences if their baby is abnormal.

'I have heard the rumors,' he sighs, 'and I can't say that I'm surprised. When man is fumbling at the source of life, not even a brilliant physician as Dr. Steptoe can read the consequences in advance.'

This implantation of Mrs. Brown was a shot in the dark, as Dr. Steptoe and Dr. Edwards both have said.

'I have said all along that if Mrs. Brown were brought to full term, that the baby was likely to be abnormal. True, I felt that a physical deformity

was most likely, or perhaps retardation.

'But super-normal power also is an abnormality. If it is true that the Brown baby has this quality, one of two things likely will happen: The child will have to be put away, or it will die very early in life because its own brain power will not permit it to live.'

Of course all this is complete and utter nonsense. Nobody in my family can remember anyone called George Landingham being part of the Daily Mail crew and if he did exist then he had a very vivid imagination. I must admit it would have been very useful if I had been born with superhuman powers to move objects with my mind and as a child I would have loved to have been able to move my toys around just by looking at them. The article is strange in that it calls Dad Gilbert - a sure sign that it didn't come from anyone that had spent any time with him.

There was certainly not a whole string of eminent brain experts making their way to our home. As I have already said the medics were keen to test everything about me to check I was normal but these were all carried out at the hospital. In fact as I grew up there were very few checks on me to see if I was any different to anyone else. I had the usual tests that everyone born at that time had as they went through their childhood.

The interesting array of doctors named in this piece couldn't have been that good as I've looked them up on the internet and none merit a mention anywhere. They have some pretty peculiar names that you would think would come up in a search engine in something other than this piece of trash about me and my family. It was rubbish like this by ignorant idiots that caused problems for my family, fueling others to believe their tall tales.

Various people in different parts of the world claimed to have messages from Jesus or from the Virgin Mary condemning Edwards and Steptoe and my Mum and Dad. Others claimed I was some sort of lucky charm and that by touching me women who had previously been unable to get pregnant could suddenly find themselves able to have a baby.

All this meant that the Catholic Church was immediately under pressure to say something about my birth and to give some guidance to religious people across the world, who were confused at the rights and wrongs of the situation.

The Catholic Archdiocese of New York called the process of IVF "morally objectionable" saying that it turned the marital bed into a "chemistry set". The Rev William Smith, a theologian and professor of moral theology at St Joseph's Seminary, New York said that the Pope had denounced the "artificial insemination" process as long ago as the 1950s.

Father Smith was one of a number of religious leaders who weren't informed enough about the difference between IVF and artificial insemination. He said the process: "may be standard in breeding horses or in botany but in a marital union we think there is something wrong with it. And what should be done with the mistakes, the genetic disorders resulting from the test-tube process? For example if everything was not turning out perfectly would we abort? The church is opposed to abortion."

It was a tough question for the Catholic Church. My birth was on July 25 and by a strange coincidence exactly 10 years earlier on July 25 1968 the Church had published Humanae Vitae, which was Latin for "Of Human Life".

Pope Paul VI had been the author of this important document for the church, which had set out views and guidance for people on the subject of having babies. It had the subtitle "On the regulation of birth" and it had been the Church's answer to all the moral questions being thrown up in the Swinging Sixties and the advent of the oral contraceptive pill.

People were using condoms and The Pill to control when they had babies and the church felt this was interfering with the natural will of God. Of course the ability to have sex without a baby being the result had led to many people having sex outside of marriage and the church also disapproved of this.

Although the document was most famous for its views on contraception and the pill - telling Catholics that they shouldn't use it, Humanae Vitae also made reference to how far doctors should go in interfering with the natural cycle of women and how much they could use medical science to help people have babies.

Of course in 1968 nobody could predict what Steptoe and Edwards were going to achieve ten years later but the document clearly set out that it was not morally right for doctors to interfere with the natural way that people became pregnant - certainly taking an egg out of a woman and making a baby in a test-tube was interfering in a big way.

I guess we shall never know if Edwards and Steptoe were aware of the significance of the date of my birth to the church - Mum certainly had no idea that it was exactly 10 years since the Catholic pronouncement. Conspiracy theorists will no doubt conclude that the doctors induced Mum deliberately at that time to take on the church - but I'm not aware of anything like that being the case.

Pope Paul VI had suffered himself at the hands of the media for his pronouncements and some people even within the church criticised him for not coming to terms with modern thinking on sex and marriage. But in a strange way his views weren't that much different to Mum and Dad. The Pope had always said that babies should be part of a loving family with parents that were devoted to them.

Mum and Dad really believed in the idea of a family too. It was something they had been denied as children. They wanted to have a family of their own that they had created between them. They just needed the help of medical science to make that possible. They certainly believed in marriage before having babies and they were devoted to each other all their lives.

Dad said little in the debate that was now raging, preferring to let all the arguments about morals and religion be held by the religious leaders and politicians. But he did tell one reporter: "If God hadn't wanted this to happen then he wouldn't have given Steptoe and Edwards the skill to do it."

People wanted to know what Pope Paul VI had to say about my birth but sadly he was unwell and in the last few days of his life. He was being looked after away from the Vatican in his Papal Summer Residence. He died on August 6 just days after I was born. The Catholic Church had the challenge of finding a replacement and it was the soon-to-be John Paul I, who at the time was Patriarch of Venice who replied to the clamour for an opinion on my birth.

He said that people should not condemn my Mum and Dad as they had simply wanted to have a baby and that people should be sympathetic to them. He also said that he was sure God would find a place in heaven for me.

His comments about us as a family were really helpful and calmed some of the more extreme feelings against us. He was tougher on the doctors and the IVF pioneers, questioning whether artificial conception would produce more malformed children and saying they were unleashing things that they could not control.

He also said that it could be used in the future to "manufacture" babies for people who were not married, hinting at single parenthood and same sex marriages, which of course were unthinkable in 1978. He said these things would be a great setback for society and for families.

Because they were not as expected his comments about our family were the most widely reported and were helpful to Mum and Dad, even though they no doubt upset those who wanted those close to the Pope to say that my birth was evil and I was some sort of Satanic figure. It meant that the extremists with their strident religious views got some sensible guidance from Rome. But hang on - how weird was that - I am just days old living in an ordinary house in the backstreets of Bristol, England and my very existence is being debated by those close to the Pope and causing shockwaves around the world.

Other religions also had their say. Rabbi Siegel, professor of ethics at the Jewish Theological Seminary in New York, told reporters: "My

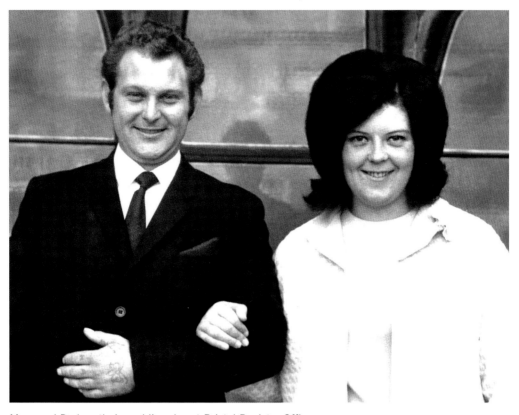

Mum and Dad on their wedding day at Bristol Register Office. © Family collection

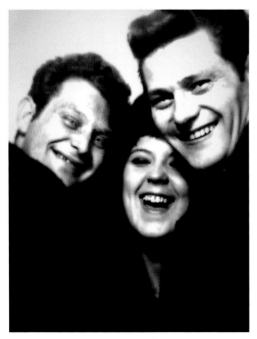

Mum and Dad in a photobooth picture with another friend in their days at The Holborn.

© Family collection

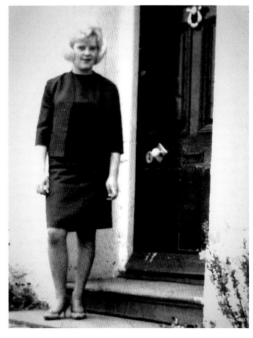

Mum with the peroxide blonde hairstyle that marked her teenage rebellion. © Family collection

Dear Mrs. Brown,

Thank you for your letter, I shall of course be pleased to see you and your husband and can offer you an appointment on Thursday 6th July at 10.45 a.m. However, after an operation such as yours, obviously you must realise that the chances of anything being done are not very great.

With best wishes,

Yours sincerely,

Dr. R. A. Hinton
Medical Officer to the
Female Sub-fertility Clinic.

The first letter after Mum asked for help held out little hope. © Family collection

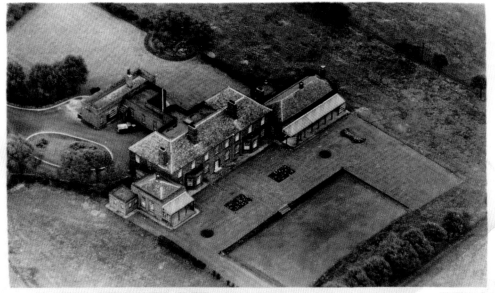

DR. KERSHAW'S COTTAGE HOSPITAL, ROYTON   CA.229A

A postcard of Dr Kershaw's Hospital where the IVF took place. Jean Purdy and Bob Edwards wrote their home addresses and numbers on this for Mum to keep in touch. © Family collection

Physiological Laboratory
Downing Street
Cambridge
CB2 3EG

December 6th., 1977

Dear Mrs Brown,

Just a short note to let you know that the early results on your blood and urine samples are very encouraging, and indicate that you might be in early pregnancy.

So please take things quietly - no skiing, climbing, or anything too strenuous including Xmas shopping!

If you should wish to get in touch with me for any reason before seeing Mr Steptoe next week, my laboratory number is ███████, and my home number is ███████. Best wishes.

Yours sincerely,

[signature]

Dr R. G. Edwards.

The letter that Dad opened telling Mum she was pregnant – Bob Edwards guessed she would be Christmas shopping. © Family collection

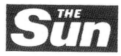

Registered Office
30 Bouverie Street,
Fleet Street,
London, EC4Y 8DE.
Telephone: 01-353 3030
Telegraphic Address
Sunfleet Ldn, EC4
Telex Sunnews Ldn, 267827
Registered No. 679215 England

News Group Newspapers Ltd.
A Subsidiary of News International Ltd.

MANCHESTER OFFICE:
G.P.O. Box 294
1-23 Withy Grove,
Manchester 4
Telephone 061-834 1234

Thursday April 27

Dear Mr Brown,
      We can't go on meeting like this!
      All I wanted to ask you this morning
was whether or not you had received my first letter.
      I also wanted to draw your attention to the
enclosed article from yesterday's 'Daily Mail' as an
indication of the amount of interest in this story.
      As I said in my previous note I only
want to get you to listen to what I have to say.
      My paper would like an interview with
you and Lesley about your hopes and feelings at this
time.
      You have my absolute assurance that you
would NOT be named or identified in any way.
      In return we would reward you with a
substantial financial payment which perhaps you would
like to use as a deposit for a home of your own or
for whatever purpose you decide.
      I beg you—at least listen to what I have
to say. If you are still uncertain then perhaps I could
meet your father or father in law whenever or
wherever you like and they could pass the details on.
      I am now staying at the Holiday Inn. Tel:
Bristol 294281. If you or a relative could ring me
this evening at 7.30pm or later at your convenience I
would be happy to come and outline my proposals.
      The last thing I want is to cause distress
for you or your family so you have nothing to fear or
to lose by listening to what I have to say.
      Again sincere best wishes,

Charles A Garside.

Charles Garside. Staff Reporter.

Three months before my birth and The Sun newspaper had dispatched a reporter to Bristol to try to sign up the family for an "exclusive" story. The reporter was living in a nearby hotel © Family collection.

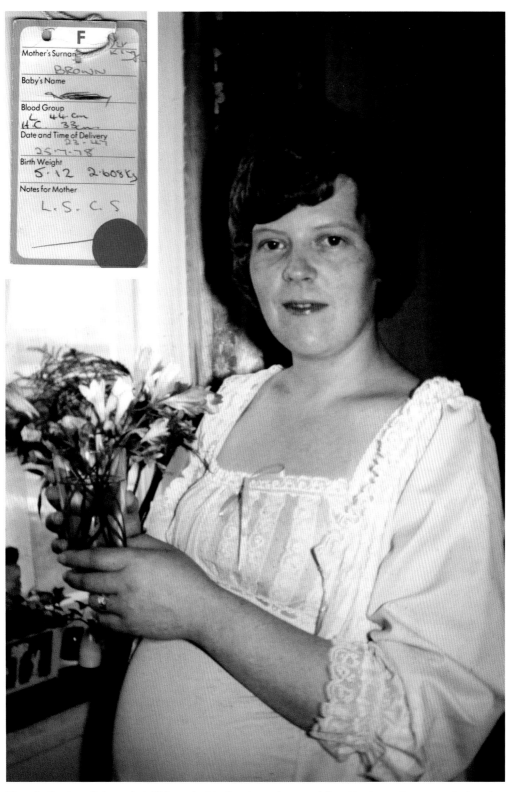

Mum in the hospital ward at Oldham just before I was born and (inset) a tag put on my cot when I was born © Family collection

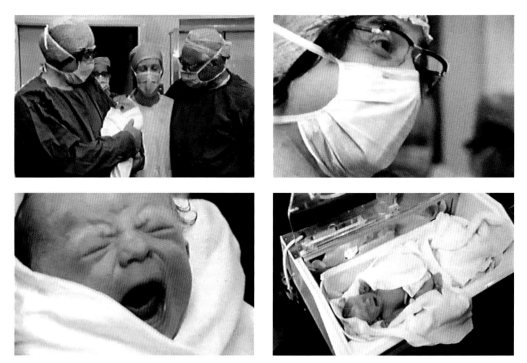

Scenes from the Central Office of Information film of my birth, showing the proud team of Bob Edwards, Jean Purdy and Patrick Steptoe with me (top left) Bob Edwards (top right) and my first few seconds of life © TV stills

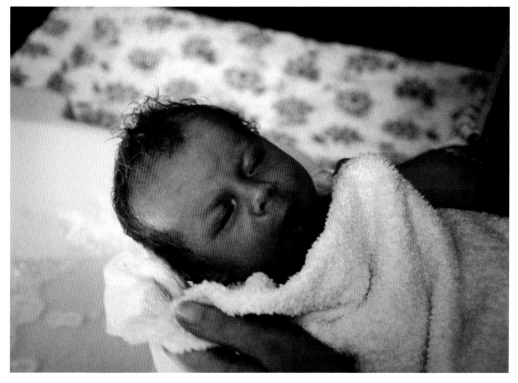

At last Mum and Dad had the baby that they wanted so much © Family collection

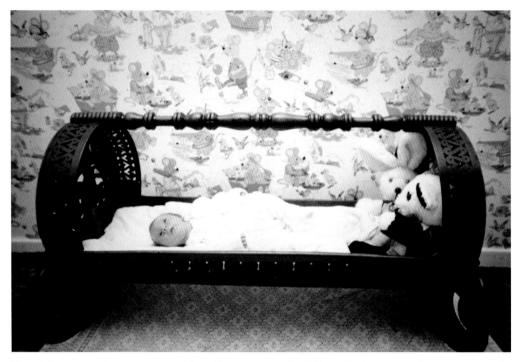

The elaborate cot that was sent to Mum "from the people of Turkey" when news of my birth spread around the world © Family collection

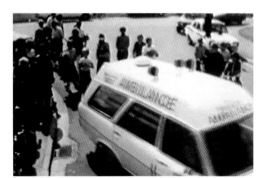

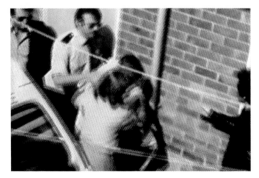

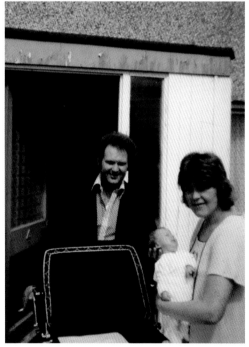

The chaotic arrival back in Bristol as crowds of reporters and the public gathered in the street and Mum and I were rushed into the house. Right: Outside the front door at Hassell Drive where the family was under siege from the world's media © TV stills and Family collection

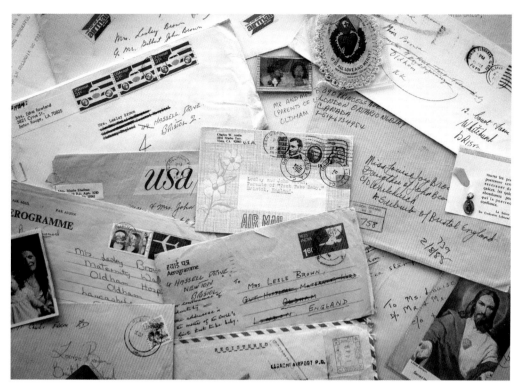

Letters came from all over the world. Even those addressed to "Test Tube Baby New York" or Louise Brown, UK got through to Mum and Dad. © Neil Phillips

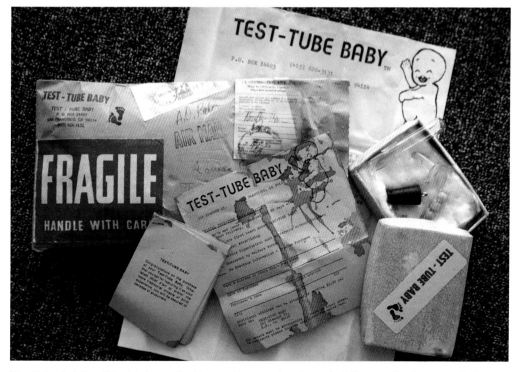

The "blood-stained" test-tube sent addressed to me when I was just five months from people in California opposed to IVF. © Neil Phillips

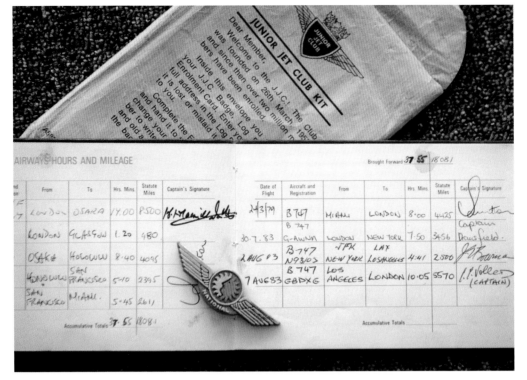

AIRWAYS HOURS AND MILEAGE

Brought Forward **37 55** *18 081*

From	To	Hrs. Mins	Statute Miles	Captain's Signature	Date of Flight	Aircraft and Registration	From	To	Hrs. Mins	Statute Miles	Captain's Signature
LONDON	OSAKA	14.00	8500	*H. Hamilton*	24/3/79	B 747	MIAMI	LONDON	8.00	4425	*Hunter Captain*
LONDON	GLASGOW	1.20	480		30.7.83	G-AWNN B 747	LONDON	NEW YORK	7.50	3456	*Dransfield*
OSAKA	HONOLULU	8.40	4095		2 AUG 83	B 747 N93103	NEW YORK JFK	LOS ANGELES LAX	4:41	2500	*J.B. Bourne*
HONOLULU	SAN FRANCISCO	5.10	2395		7 AUG 83	B 747 G BDXG	LOS ANGELES	LONDON	10.05	5570	*I.P. Vallee (CAPTAIN)*
SAN FRANCISCO	MIAMI	5.45	2611								
		Accumulative Totals	**37 55** *18 081*					Accumulative Totals			

I was enrolled into the Junior Jet Club by British Airways as a frequent flyer while still a baby. © Neil Phillips

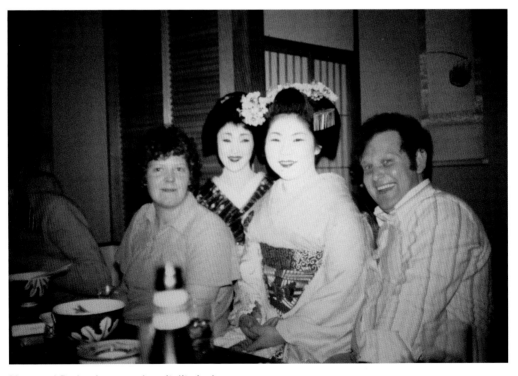

Mum and Dad enjoy some hospitality in Japan © Family collection

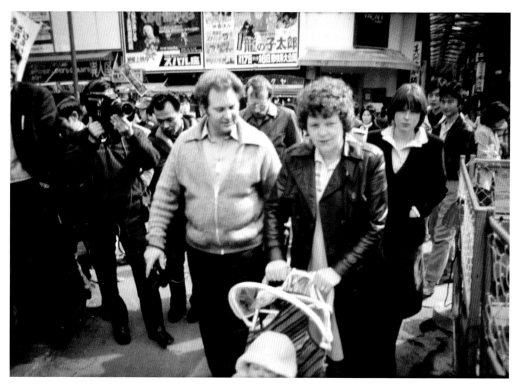

Everywhere we went in Japan crowds of people and media followed trying to get a view of me.
© Family collection

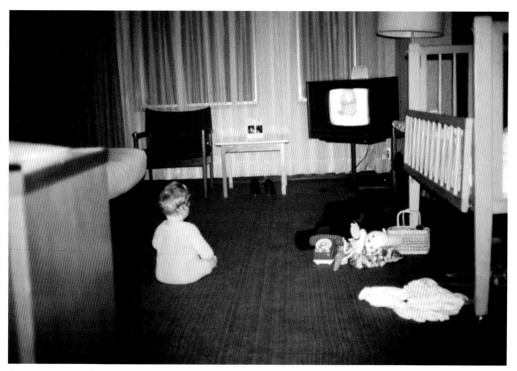

A quiet moment in a Japanese hotel room. Mum took this of me watching Patrick Steptoe on television. © Family collection

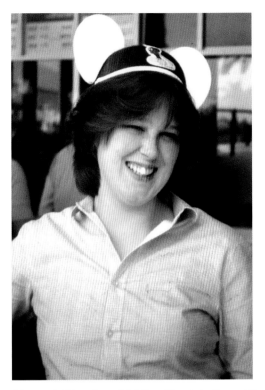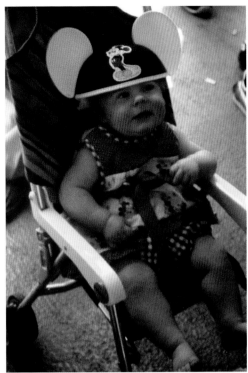

Sharon (left) and me (right) getting into the spirit of our visit to Disneyland. © Family collection

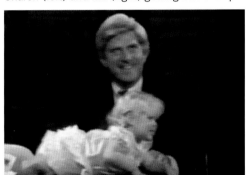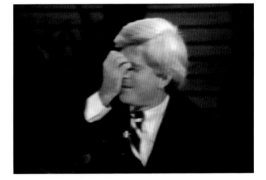

Donahue found coping with my antics a bit too much on his programme. © TV stills

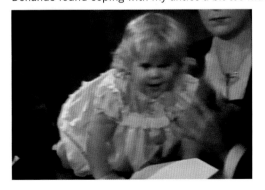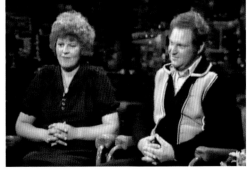

Scenes from two more American television interviews during our month long book tour. © TV stills

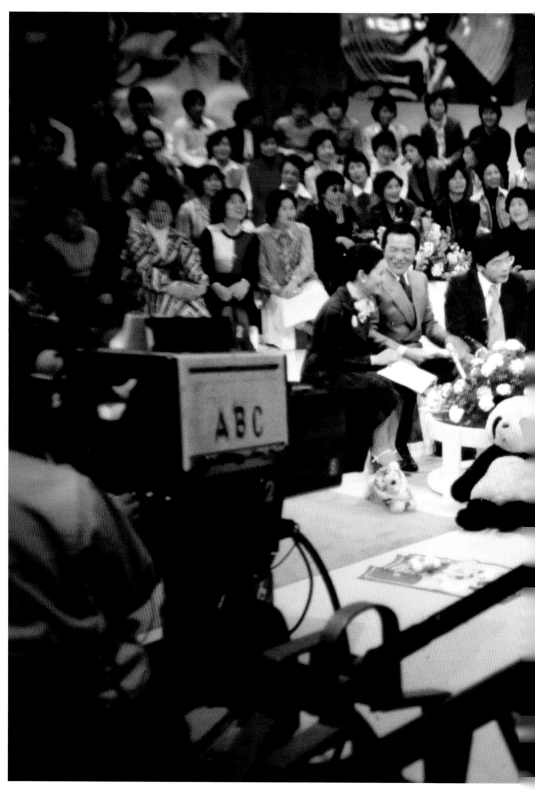

A daunting prospect for the family as we were interviewed on an Asahi Broadcasting
Company programme in Japan watched by a panel of 100 Japanese women © Family collection

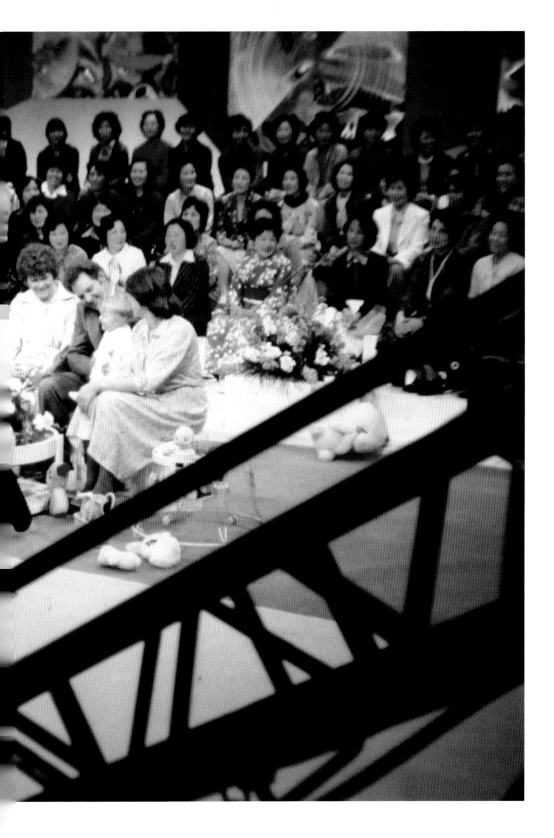

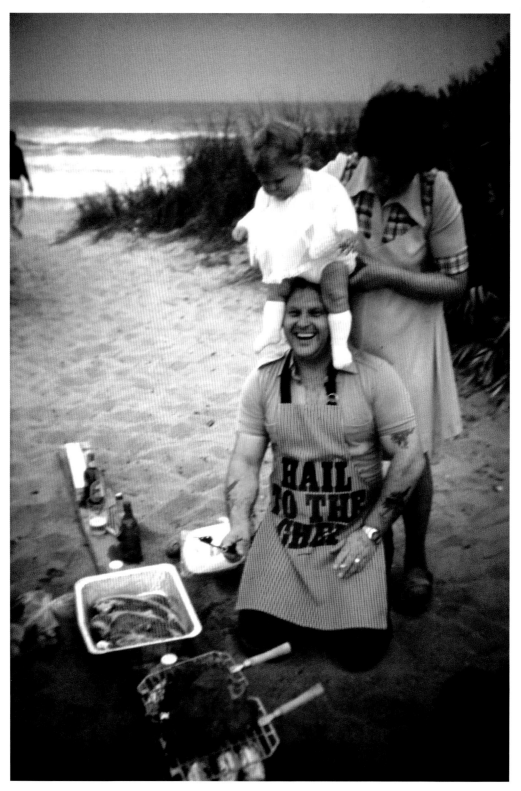

Dad cooked a barbecue during one of the few moments of down-time on the US tour. © Family collection

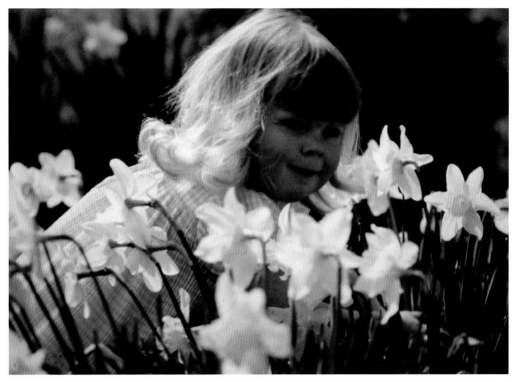

Enjoying the sunshine and flowers in our lovely garden in Whitchurch © Family collection

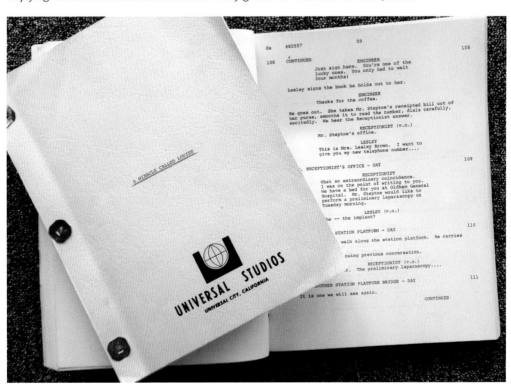

The story of my conception and birth prompted plans for a Hollywood movie. The idea was scrapped following a strike. © Neil Phillips

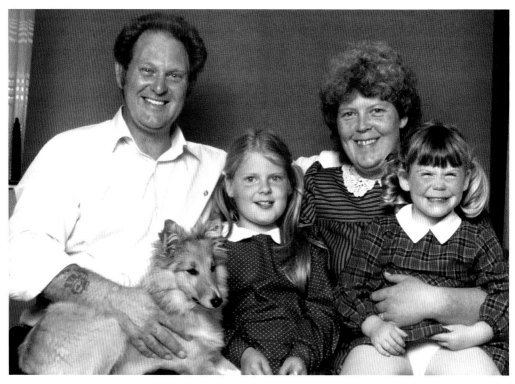

A family portrait with my sister Natalie. © Family collection

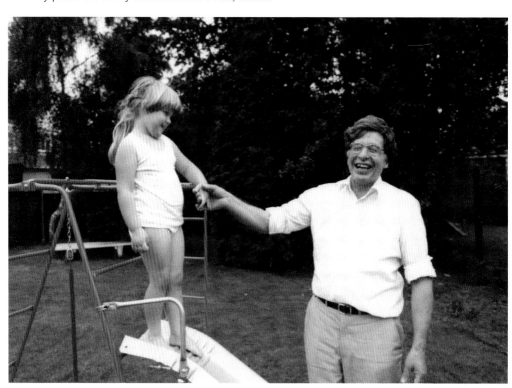

Me and Bob Edwards, who I regarded as a Grandfather figure © Bourn Hall

personal view is there is nothing wrong in the procedure. I think there is nothing wrong in trying to outwit nature which made it impossible by the accepted methods for this woman to conceive."

It became a subject for debate at religious conferences all over the world. A 12-man committee of the US Episcopal Church met to discuss my birth and the United Methodist Church had a meeting in Washington to decide on their line to take - representing over nine million Methodists in the USA.

All I was interested in at that stage was getting some milk, having a cry and dirtying my nappy and yet eminent philosophers, religious figures, journalists, professors and heads of state were busy worrying about how I might change the world. Mum and Dad couldn't really care less either about all this stuff going on. They had the baby that they wanted - somehow Steptoe and Edwards had done it - and they just wanted to get on with being ordinary parents.

Of course the religious people also had a problem about the fact that my Dad had given a sample of sperm to enable me to be conceived - and there is only one way to get that. It is always a bit embarrassing even today for the men who have to go through IVF. They have to masturbate to successfully supply the sample and that leads to a lot of jokes, nudges and winks.

This sort of activity had also been criticised by the Catholic Church. The most fundamental Christians believed that any sort of sexual activity was only permissible if it was for the purpose of having a baby - definitely not on if it was just for pleasure.

Questions were asked about this and eventually it was decreed that because Dad was masturbating in order to have a baby then that was alright in the eyes of the church. He hadn't committed any kind of sin when he was wanking into that jar - and that's official!

I think the use of the word "miracle" a lot around the time of my birth was one of the reasons that so many religious people were upset by my birth. The word was bandied about by the media and Mum and Dad were happy to let it happen because they had been given so little hope of having a child of their own that truly what Steptoe and Edwards had achieved seemed like a miracle to them.

But they didn't realise that the word would upset some people of faith in other parts of the world who believed that only God or some divine power could truly carry out miracles and that by using the word somehow Mum and Dad and the doctors were insulting their beliefs.

Back at home the Daily Mail journalist Lynda Lee-Potter interviewed Mum and Dad for another major feature to go with the pictures they had taken of us at home.

Dad told her of their plans for me: "There will be no frills. If she's got ability then she can go to college but she'll get no preferences, no easy money. She'll work for what she gets. She'll earn every penny she spends. She's going to be an ordinary girl brought up in an ordinary house as an ordinary person. If we treated her any different from Sharon, it would be wrong. When Sharon was at school and she wanted a bit of spending money she got a Saturday job in a greengrocers.

"If children are pampered all it brings is sadness. Obviously we'll show her all the photographs and tell her everything that happened as she gets older. But what I'm hoping is that by the time she goes to school there'll be hundreds like her.

"I feel half proud and half fearful. I'm frightened of anybody hurting her. I'm humble as well, to think that the implant should have worked first time for an ordinary couple like us."

I think Mum and Dad pretty much stuck to their word on that and it is a true reflection of how they always behaved towards me and Sharon in those early years.

Of course that's not how some of the other newspapers portrayed things. Unable to talk to Mum and Dad face to face and jealous of the fact that the Daily Mail had exclusive access and would only let others - like the National Enquirer - meet up with Mum and Dad if they paid; they painted a picture of a grasping, mercenary family.

Amazingly the coverage in the newspapers led to a huge influx of letters from all over the world. The Post Office did an amazing job -

letters addressed in Australia to "Mrs. Lesley Brown, Maternity Ward, Oldham Hospital, England" arrived at Hassell Drive; letters from America simply addressed "Louise Brown, Test-tube Baby, Bristol, England" got to us. Mum saved all the letters she received in this avalanche of mail.

Many letters were from women who couldn't have babies. One woman from Christchurch, New Zealand, wrote with her story of operations that hadn't worked, treatments that had failed and her desire to be a Mum. She pleaded with Mum to pass her details on to Edwards and Steptoe in case they could help. That was a common theme from all over the world - mothers that saw some hope in my Mum's story and my birth.

Addressed to "Gilbert John Brown" at Oldham Hospital came a letter from Ontario, Canada from a woman proud of her four adopted children but keen to know if the procedure Mum had could help her.

From West Bengal came a letter from a man asking curiously for photographs of me and Dad so that he could compare how we looked and asking if he could come to see us.

A woman in Nawalapitiya, Sri Lanka wrote to say she had a baby girl on the same day so wanted to compare notes with Mum as the babies grew up. From Calcutta came a letter from a man asking Mum for the air fare so that he could fly to "the great city of London" as he had always wanted to visit but couldn't afford it.

Heather Spackman from New South Wales, Australia wrote: "I fear that you will find yourselves on the receiving end of all the usual criticism and condemnation that follows any medical breakthrough, so am writing to try in a tiny way to even things up.

"A lot of people throughout the world will be grateful to you, and I hope that you will remember that at any time that criticism 'gets you down'. Thank you for making public what you have done, and thereby giving hope to thousands of would-be parents. I'm sure that Katrina will bring you great happiness. Despite all the sleepless nights, wet nappies and tantrums there's no joy like that of watching and helping a child grow up!"

Lovely sentiments and there were more letters of support than condemnation - but who the hell is Katrina? I can only suppose that was another mistake in a newspaper on the other side of the world!

Other letters came from religious people criticising Mum for praising the medics. They said she should "let God have the glory" and saying that she should ensure that the baby is brought up to love God and believe in Christ.

From Devonport came a letter from an 84-year-old Great Grannie, who had seen my photo in the paper and asked Mum to give me a kiss from her; another elderly lady called Queenie from Devon wrote saying that "I am not given to writing to strangers but this is a very very special request." She wanted Mum to change my name to Patricia Louise Roberta in honour of the doctors as a "gesture of everlasting record to the work of the two men."

Little religious texts and booklets came all the time. Little medals with pictures of Jesus and the Virgin Mary arrived from around the world. One person drew around their hand on a piece of paper and wrote across the top: "this hand is 63 years old" they then wrote underneath: "I am only Jesus friend, wash our Louise feet; now 29th July 1978. Time now is 1 O'clock AM. I am going to bed now. God Bless". This was accompanied by several pages of quotes from the Bible and bits from a calendar on the day I was born with random quotes from the book of Proverbs on them.

I don't quite know how Mum coped with this stuff pouring through the letterbox every day; the constant media knocks on the door alongside the usual difficulties of trying to look after your first baby.

Then there were the autograph hunters. Dozens of people from all over the world sent things for Mum to sign. She and Dad did sign some and send them back. Many were from stamp collectors who wanted signatures on stamps issued on the day I was born.

Then there were the astrologers with their charts of how the stars were lined up the moment I was born and what it might mean for my future.

The London Evening Standard astrologer Katina outlined my future: "The child's horoscope shows good artistic potential and this will probably influence her choice of career. She also has the makings of a very successful business woman. Money will come her way easily and she will invest it shrewdly especially in land or property."

All I can say is I'm still waiting for that to happen! Other astrologers sent incomprehensible charts drawn in the fashionable felt pens of the time. Some other astrologers wrote asking Mum to send them the time, date and place of my birth - which considering those facts had been in newspapers all around the world didn't fill you with confidence in the fact that they might have fantastic powers of foretelling the future!

Also entertaining for the family when they arrived were the dozens of letters from all over the world with some excuse or another for a photograph to be sent. It became pretty clear straight away that these letters were in fact from journalists keen to get an "exclusive" who thought that by posing as a little old lady or someone with a disability they might get a photo that they would be able to make money on without having to pay for a photo from the Daily Mail.

A constant stream of letters from journalists arrived all pretty much saying the same thing, they just wanted a brief interview, it would take just a few minutes and they would only concentrate on upbeat and positive issues. What none of them seemed to realise is that it was impossible to grant all the requests just because of the sheer number of media enquiries coming in from all over the world - plus what else could Mum and Dad say. Their story had now been told all over the world. They had a baby. They were happy. They just wanted people to go away!

Still the letters and requests were pouring through the letterbox every day. Early in September a letter and brochure arrived from a company called Cindico. They had written to Mum originally the day after I was born saying that their baby products were used by Princess

Anne, Anthea Forsyth (then wife of Bruce Forsyth), Lulu and Esther Rantzen! They were following up that letter, which not surprisingly Mum had not really read it properly.

In fact they wanted to give Mum a folding pushchair and this time they didn't wait for her to ask for it - they just sent it! Mum was keen to try it out and really wanted to go out for a walk with it. But there was almost always some journalist or another lurking by the gate. Mum hadn't been out of doors with her new baby yet.

One day Mum just put me in the new pram and went out for the first time. She was just going to cross the road when she saw two men wearing long belted macs and she realised reporters were following her. She ran back home with the pram in panic. The siege was continuing.

When they told the Daily Mail about the problem they arranged for a little trip to the countryside – but of course it included a photographer to capture the event for the first time. Then they arranged a little trip into Bristol, again with a photographer, which just attracted attention from passing shoppers.

The main reason for the continued press siege was the fact that people all over the world wanted to know more and more about Mum and Dad. That was clear from the letters from people - most of whom just wanted to reach out and say something about their own lives and their own struggle to have children.

Dad was persuaded that one way to relieve that pressure would be to do a book deal and a journalist and writer called Sue Freeman spent some time with Mum and Dad recording their memories of their lives to date on a tape recorder. The idea was to bring the book out with profits going into Chandlewise to top up the company money. Mum and Dad were still getting paid out at £250 a month.

Certain people at Dad's workplace weren't very happy about some of the time he had taken off - there was no paternity leave in those days and men couldn't even have one day off when a baby was born. Because of the trips to Oldham he'd used up his holidays and even took some unpaid days off. Some supervisors and managers were putting pressure on him - so he was delighted when he got a letter from Sir Peter Parker, Chairman of the British Railways Board and the ultimate boss. It congratulated him on my birth and wished him well. Good ammunition for shutting up the local managers who were on his back! In fact as soon as he could he got back into the swing of work. Dad just wanted everything to be normal again.

But there was little chance of that. After all, what other working class family in Bristol or anywhere else were front page news all around the world - receiving stacks of mail every day, receiving requests for radio and television interviews every day and booking sessions with a writer who was putting together their biography.

All through those first few weeks of my life one song was dominating the pop charts - John Travolta and Olivia Newton-John singing "You're the one that I want"...there couldn't be a more appropriate song for Mum to sing along to her new born baby that she had wanted so much. But now I was here I seemed to have brought a whole bundle of trouble with me in the form of this worldwide interest!

Chapter 5

POEMS, HEADLINES
AND TV SHOWS

The number of journalists waiting fruitlessly outside the house gradually dwindled but the letters and parcels from every corner of the globe kept arriving at the little house in the middle of Bristol. Every aspect of the family was proving fascinating for people.

Sharon was seventeen and had appeared in some of the pictures. As well as letters from potential boyfriends she got media requests from as far away as Tokyo - where the Japanese magazine called Shosetsu Junior wanted to interview her about being my sister and to "talk to her about her feelings and her teenage life in general."

From 20-year-old Farhad Phiroze Hotelwaha in Bombay, India came a letter in beautiful copperplate handwriting wishing Mum and Dad the best of luck.

He said: "I want to suggest one thing. You may be knowing about the famous lovers Shirin and Farhad. A long way back in Persia there were two great lovers Shirin and Farhad. As my name is Farhad I request you to name your baby Shirin. I came to know that you have a 17 year old daughter by your previous marriage whose name is Sharon. The name of the pair Sharon and Shirin will sound very beautiful."

To be honest I'm not sure having two children called Sharon and Shirin works very well in a Bristol accent but the fact that someone so far away was coming up with a suggestion was an indication of just how crazy things were getting for the family.

Little oil paintings and drawings arrived where people had either imagined what I looked like or produced a painting inspired by the smudged black and white photograph they had seen in their newspaper. Then there was a whole clutch of poems.

Mr A.E Sperrin of Lichfield, Staffordshire sent Mum and Dad a poem with a note saying that he had also copied it to the Queen who he said had accepted much of his poetical works over the 25 years of her reign to that date.

In eight verses he summed up the process of IVF. The fourth verse has the fantastic opening line, which Wordsworth could never have written: "A month passed and menstruation did not appear to Mrs Brown's delight and her husband too".

The last two verses read:

"People of all nations had waited expectantly
For the good news of the miracle babies birth.
In Oldham General Hospital the staff in Maternity
Unit had made preparations right down to earth,
And a superb cot was ready for the babies berth (sic).
Medical staff were waiting as the time drew near,
There was a feeling of triumph in the atmosphere.

By Caesarian birth little Louise Brown was born,
The first test-tube baby to be born alive.
With blue eyes, and fair hair her young head to adorn,
She was beautiful, normal and should she survive
She was wealthy now, so there would be no need to strive.
Proud were the two parents delighted were all,
Especially the Doctor pioneers who answered the call,
That call of the childless, upon deaf-ears did not fall.

Another poem from Barbara L Grant from Glasgow, Scotland came along with a hand-written note pondering on whether caesarian or cesarean is the correct spelling and ending with the true words to Mum: "I don't suppose this will worry you much as you know what it really means".

Her poem in full was:

Louise Brown
of world renown
Born the Caesarian Way
Arrived upon a Tuesday

A babe indeed
Born from a seed
Planted a different way
delivered neither early or late.

Transferred in time
At a given sign
To grow by nature engendered
By Science carefully rendered.

Nurtured and grown
Once it was sown
Like a plant in a gardener's frame
In all its beauty it came.

A wonder child:
As any child
produced by every mother
Unique, unlike another.

A ray of hope
To those who mope
Upon their barren state
Now may calmly wait.

A child in the making
if not world shaking
A miracle in its entirety
Individuals of every variety.

In September a parcel arrived and inside was a lovely little dress for me. Also enclosed was a clipping from a newspaper with an article about Mum.

The covering letter was from world famous cartoonist Kim Casali, who by then was living in a mansion in Weybridge, Surrey following the success of her "Love is..." cartoons that had been syndicated in newspapers worldwide and were used on millions of greetings cards, calendars and posters in the 1970s.

In 1975 her husband Roberto had been diagnosed with testicular cancer. They had two sons, Stefano and Dario. Kim so wanted to have a little girl to complete the family and with the devastating news of her husband's diagnosis feared she wouldn't get pregnant before her husband died. The pair agreed to store some sperm in December 1975 and sadly Roberto died in March 1976.

Despite opposition from many people around the world Kim bravely went ahead with artificial insemination treatment at a clinic in Cambridge and in July 1977 - a year before I entered the world - her son Milo Roberto Andrea Casali weighed in at 10lb 8 oz.

Controversy raged. He was described as a "miracle baby" as he had been conceived seven months after his father had died. The Vatican said that the act by Kim had been "immoral" and there were debates in Parliament about whether the baby would have the right to inherit the wealth of the family as his father had died before he was conceived...a question to make more lawyers rich.

His Mum had only really been able to push through the treatment because she had made so much money from her cartoons and that also prompted criticism from ignorant people around the world saying it was something only rich people could do - this was despite the fact that she had many years in poverty before her talents had made her successful.

Kim Casali announced the birth with a special "Love is..." cartoon of a girl pushing a pram. The press had a field day and Kim did the same as Mum and Dad did a year later - seeking the protection of the Daily Mail. Her letter to Mum was timely from one Mum who had been through a lot to another. It read:

"Congratulations for having such a beautiful daughter. I do admire your determination to overcome the drawbacks you must have faced in order to have your own child. I hope the Daily Mail is looking after you well as they looked after me. We are all very good friends whereas two of the other newspapers were deliberately unkind and caused me considerable anguish.

"I am enclosing a clipping which was from a Canadian or American paper. It was sent to me because there was an article about me on the same page. I've taken no notice of the religious criticisms of the method I used to get the baby I wanted so much. Usually the people who criticise are people who have absolutely no idea of what it is like to desperately want a baby.

"I am also enclosing a little dress. I bought it in Holland before I had even conceived Milo. I thought it was very sweet and I wanted a girl so badly I bought it anyway. I was hoping I was pregnant at the time but it took me six treatments. Anyway I have another son and so I thought the little dress might suit Louise. All the very best for the future."

It must have been quite a big decision for Kim Casali to give away that little dress as the final act of coming to terms with the fact that she had been blessed with sons. No doubt seeing all the reports in the paper just a year after her own time in the spotlight prompted the act. Sadly Kim Casali succumbed to cancer herself in 1996 after raising her three sons. Her cartoons live on giving pleasure to millions.

In October an Air Mail parcel arrived addressed simply to "Louise Brown, Test-tube Baby, Bristol, England" it had been posted in San Francisco and the customs' sticker on it said it contained a novelty item.

Inside Mum found a small jewellery-style box with the words "Test-tube Baby" printed on a sticker with an image of some baby footprints.

She thought maybe it was another gift from a corporate anxious to be associated with my birth but when she opened it there was red liquid that looked as if it had spilled and a carefully folded letter.

The letter was signed Marjorie K Little, Edy Potts, Alex Mexi and Anthony Cassinelli. It was addressed to me and said:

"Dear Louise, By the time you receive this, you should be nearly three months old. Your birth was a tremendous inspiration to us. Most children have only dolls and stuffed animals to play with. We feel it is only right that you should have your own TEST-TUBE BABY. Because it was issued in a month with an "R" in it you can be assured it is also a little girl. We haven't given her a name. We thought we'd leave that up to you. The Normalettes will be in England next month and hope to meet up with you and your family."

The next piece of paper again spattered in red ink to look like blood was a "Test-tube baby" warranty card then a little typewritten booklet with sick little questions and answers. One suggesting that you could keep a test-tube baby in a toilet bowl or fish tank. Another suggesting that you could buy a turkey baster to help you insert a test-tube baby into the womb.

It ends with a page that says: "Where do test-tube babies come from? Ans: Ask your mother." Beneath this was a piece of cotton wool and below that a broken and jagged glass test-tube and finally lying in the bottom a plastic baby foetus.

It was menacing and scary and considering the time the people must have taken in putting this thing together then sending it across the world to a three month old baby I would say a completely sick act by some sick minds.

Imagine how worrying this was for Mum, especially with the vague threat that "the Normalettes" were on their way to England to "meet up". For a while she was even more careful when taking me out in the pram.

A television crew came and did a documentary on the family called: "To Mrs Brown, a daughter." They filmed me being fed by Mum and Dad in our little house and showed the family going about its normal business. It helped to show people that we were just normal working class people, but with just three main channels on British television it was watched by a huge chunk of the country and simply sparked off a whole new load of post and fuss just as everything was dying down.

Somehow, despite all the fuss going on around them, Mum and Dad managed to carry on as normally as possible. I was getting bigger every day and although the rows still rumbled on about whether test-tube babies were morally right, whether cheque-book journalism was a bad thing or not and almost daily someone beat a path to their door asking for an interview or a comment Dad went back to work and Mum settled down to looking after her baby.

For some reason - I suspect because somebody in authority was causing problems - Mum was asked to take me to the local hospital in Bristol for a check up from the top baby doctor in the area. He, once again, pronounced me perfectly normal. I'm not sure what they were looking for but it was the last time that anyone seemed to question whether having babies by IVF produced anything other than a perfectly normal baby that was the same as a baby conceived by normal means.

Sue Freeman made good progress with the book and Mum and Dad were given copies of the words she had written. It was to be called "Our Miracle Called Louise - A parents' story" and Sue Freeman had written it with chapters in my Mum's words or in my Dad's words based on the tape recordings she had made of them.

Dad was always very chatty and outgoing but Mum was never particularly keen to chat to anyone and chose her words carefully. Some of the newspaper and magazine articles quoting her are quite laughable when you read them now as they don't sound much like the sort of thing Mum would say. Sue Freeman's book was a reasonable account of what had happened to Mum and Dad - obviously made a bit dramatic in places to keep people interested. They read through the proofs and the deal was sealed for the book to be published early in 1979.

Just before Christmas a deal was struck for the family to go to Toronto, Canada to appear on a Canadian discussion television programme about IVF. So, aged just four months old, I travelled across the Atlantic for the first time with my family.

Money earned went into the Chandlewise company and Paul Vincent travelled along as well to ensure everything went to plan. It was a whistle-stop trip, especially as Mum and Dad took the opportunity to also go to New York where Mum was able to meet up with an old family friend from Bristol who had married an American GI soldier and gone to live in the USA.

It was pretty amazing stuff for Mum and Dad. Just a few years before they had been sleeping rough in railway sidings in Bristol. Now, because of a simple desire to have a baby they were on all-expenses paid trips across the world visiting countries that never in their wildest dreams did they think they would see.

The first trip was a success and the family was back home for Christmas. Of course a baby's first Christmas is always special and the Daily Mail saw this as another opportunity to show me off to the world.

Dad was dressed up in a Father Christmas outfit for the photos and under the headline: "She has chubby cheeks is always laughing and the whole world sends her this wish: Happy Christmas lovely Louise!" A picture of me aged just 21 weeks was the double-page spread of the national paper.

The newspaper described how Mum and Dad had decorated the biggest Christmas tree they had ever had.

The paper said: "Already there is a huge pile of presents beneath it. There is a musical mobile, an activity centre, soft, cuddly toys, noisy toys that are pulled on a string, others that can be pushed, a locket from an American lorry driver, a mysterious looking parcel from Japan and row upon row of Christmas cards from all over the world.

"But the main present from Louise's proud parents won't fit underneath. It is a wooden rocking horse with a flowing mane and a special baby saddle."

That Christmas morning I got a wooden Snoopy dog from Sharon and a pink, fluffy pig. Dad cooked the Christmas turkey dinner and apparently we spent the day quietly at home - no media bothered us.

In their Christmas special the American National Enquirer carried the photos of me in Dad's arms - Dad dressed as Santa. The story was supposed to be written by Mum but was in fact put together by a journalist. It tells how at exactly five months old I weighed in at 14 pounds 12 ounces.

The article says: "John and I, this year, put 140 tiny lights on our Christmas tree. And when Louise saw it all aglow for the first time, her eyes opened up as big as saucers. She waved her little arms and giggled.

"John had tears in his eyes when he held her up so that she could touch the ornaments. He was so moved he couldn't talk."

In fact Dad quite often got emotional when doing interviews in that first year or so. Mum usually was matter-of-fact and calm when faced by the media questioning but often Dad had to dab a tear from his eye as he was asked to describe his feelings about having a baby of his own. He was a rough, tough man with "love" and "hate" tattooed on his knuckles and a life of hard graft behind him, but like so many other men he wanted to have a baby just as much as Mum and couldn't believe this had all happened to him.

Just after Christmas another significant event happened. In January,

1979 suddenly I wasn't the only test-tube baby in the world. Mum had read an exclusive story in the Daily Mail in November about a couple called Jimmy and Grace Montgomery. Grace was in the later stages of pregnancy having undergone treatment in the same way as Mum.

Grace, a professional cookery teacher, had been told six years earlier that she would never be able to have a baby. She and Jimmy had been childhood sweethearts attending the same school in Stirlingshire and had been friends since they were 15 years old. At the age of 32 she was willing to try anything to try to get the child they wanted and in the May - two months before I was born - she was one of 20 women to have IVF treatment in Oldham and she became pregnant. A previous attempt in February 1977 had failed.

She had seen all the fuss in the newspapers that Mum and Dad had been through. Her due date was February 14, 1979, and as the date got nearer it became clear that she was going to give birth to the second test-tube baby ever to be born in the world.

It was a very significant event for Patrick Steptoe and Robert Edwards as some doctors had cast doubt on whether I had been born in the way they said at all. Those who did said maybe it was a freak one-off event that couldn't be repeated. Patrick Steptoe had refused to rush into publishing full details of his work until he had a number of examples. This had again made those who were against IVF suspicious of his work.

By producing a second test-tube baby Steptoe and Edwards were able to prove that the technique could be a step forward for childless couples all over the world.

Alastair James Lauchlan Montgomery was born a month early in January weighing 5lb 12 oz at Stobhill Hospital, Glasgow.

Once again the Daily Mail bought the exclusive. They also organised a meeting between Mum and Grace at a hotel near Glasgow when Alastair was just three weeks old.

Our family were flown up to Scotland and photographs were taken of the two families together and at that meeting Mum and Grace became firm friends despite the miles between them - after all they were the only two women in the world at that time who had been through the experience of having an IVF baby.

Mum was able to give Grace some tips about the way the press behaved and she was able to dodge them a little. Despite the strange way that we were thrown together the two mums became life-long friends and I grew up with "Auntie" Grace, a lovely, gentle lady.

Steptoe and Edwards took the opportunity of the media attention they got from the birth of Alastair to announce to the world that they intended to set up a specialist IVF clinic in Cambridgeshire. Steptoe was now too old to work in the National Health service but there was nothing to stop him continuing to develop his expertise privately, to develop the IVF techniques further and to teach others his techniques while helping other childless couples.

The "test-tube baby" bandwagon was well and truly rolling. Mum and Dad were happy with their new family and they were certainly better off than they had ever been before. But the benefits had come at a price though, they had sacrificed their privacy and it seemed the whole world wanted a piece of their baby. If they thought the madness of 1978 would calm down they were in for a shock in 1979 as the interest in me got even more intense.

Alastair has also become a good friend over the years and the two families spent many good times together and Alastair and I have been brought together on many milestone occasions in the IVF world.

Chapter 6

WORLD TOUR: "NICE PEOPLE, BAD GUESTS"

The British Airways Boeing 747 number G-ANNF landed at Osaka Airport in Japan and taxied along the tarmac bringing to an end a 17 hour flight from London covering 8,500 miles. The captain filled out the details and signed a little blue book that the stewards were planning to take back to the passenger section and present to one of the youngest passengers on board – me! At less than eight months old, in March 1979, I was presented with flying wings and my membership of the Junior Jet Club.

Our little party consisted of Mum and Dad, Sharon and Paul Vincent. Not really understanding what was happening I had spent the last 17 hours being passed from hand to hand, wriggling, crying when my ears hurt as we descended, eating baby food spooned into my mouth by Mum and Sharon and, for four blissful hours of the journey for the adults, falling asleep on an aeroplane seat.

Everyone was pleased when the cabin doors opened and a blast of warm Japanese air flooded through the plane. Sharon was particularly keen to get off and picked me up and marched to the door of the plane. It was pouring with rain outside but the Japanese media, anxious to get a first glance of the "test-tube baby" had been allowed on to the tarmac.

Mum and Dad were still gathering bits and pieces from the overhead locker as Sharon walked down the slippery steps and straight into a melee of Japanese press people. They jostled, they pushed, people fell over - it was like a scene involving The Beatles, Bay City Rollers or Take That. But in the middle of this was an eight-month old baby held aloft by a frightened teenager.

Dad got to the door of the plane at the top of the steps and shouted at Sharon to come back but she was being mobbed by the camera people. Dad started down the steps as Mum got to the door to see her baby being jostled and her daughter barely able to stand on her feet as the mob pushed and shoved trying to get photographs. All the time they shouted, some in Japanese, some in English.

The air crew waded in and eventually Sharon managed to pass me to Dad tears in her eyes. Welcome to Japan.

Mum said it was the most scared she had been during that first year - fearing that the baby that had taken such an effort to get might be injured in the unseemly scrum.

Of course by now I was a flying veteran. We had been to Canada a few months before and in February we had flown from London to Glasgow to see the Montgomery family. But this was something very different indeed - few ordinary people in 1979 travelled to Japan and Osaka seemed an alien environment to Mum and Dad who couldn't understand the language, knew little about the culture and found it hard to come to terms with the strange food on offer. We were to spend eight days in Japan satisfying the curiosity of the Japanese people about the test-tube baby they had read about in all their papers and on their television.

Mum and Dad had been impressed with a Japanese film crew that had been to our house three weeks before and made a mini-documentary about us. They had been terrifically polite compared to the British television crews. Dad had been filmed taking his lorry out of the depot close to Temple Meads Station in the snow and driving it around Bristol.

The Japanese had also followed Mum in the snow as she took me to be weighed at the clinic and me having a bath at home. Then they had stopped people in the street in Broadmead shopping centre, Bristol to ask them what they thought of the "test-tube baby" and had stood at the bottom of Park Street, Bristol asking women if they would put themselves through IVF if they couldn't have a baby normally.

The Japanese had also gone to Oldham and filmed the bed that Mum had been in when I was born and walked through the clinic with Patrick Steptoe telling them about the success he had so far had with two babies being born and the sad story of two other women who had become pregnant through his methods but had lost their babies.

Patrick Steptoe said that his success rate was 20% at the time, which he described as "a good start".

The incident at the airport shook the whole family who were pleased to finally get to a hotel and have some rest. Mum had taken very little clothing as she had filled most of her suitcase with baby food - fearing that she wouldn't be able to get anything I would eat in Japan.

The schedule included a major television appearance and at the Asahi Broadcasting Corporation studios Mum and Dad were put into make-up along with Sharon.

The programme was in a studio with100 women all sat in rows. A male and female presenter, called Nakahara and Aikawa sat with a huge bunch of flowers in front of this massive line-up of women and introduced the subject of test-tube babies.

Mum and Dad had been supplied with an interpreter and they walked on with him to applause, Mum in a green dress carrying a handbag. I was being looked after behind the scenes by Sharon while Paul Vincent watched from the wings.

Dad told the presenter that the incident at the airport had been "frightening" but went on diplomatically to say he had been "impressed by the hospitality and the friendliness" of the people he had met.

It was a pretty awkward interview. Mum and Dad were out of their comfort zone in a big way and answered with shorter and shorter answers as they had no idea what was going on with the presenters asking in Japanese, the interpreter then repeating it in his best English and then repeating their answers back to the presenters.

There was also a lot of bowing and politeness - in stark contrast to the media scrum at the airport. They showed the film that had been taken in Britain before we flew out and finally Sharon brought me on to the set wearing a knitted yellow jumper, my hair slightly disheveled as I had been woken up from a sleep just seconds before going on.

The 100 Japanese women cooed and looked pleased and a giant panda was produced for me to play with, Dad told the audience that he needed to cut my food down as I was eating too much but that my birth had made a complete family.

Sharon, smiling nervously, looked after me in a sisterly way and I rewarded her by trying to strangle her with her own necklace as she picked me up. The programme ended with the 100 women being polled on what they thought of IVF treatment after some incomprehensible Japanese adverts for things Mum and Dad could barely understand.

The rest of the week was spent with visits to various places. Dad was impressed by the modern high speed Japanese trains and the party was treated to some meals where traditional Geisha girls attended in their costumes, organizing drinking games with Dad and Paul Vincent and Mum.

I was presented with the most beautiful silk kimono and ceremonial Japanese fan at one event and a Sumo wrestler came to our hotel room to meet me and pose for the cameras. From time to time we ventured out into the streets to have a look around but invariably within minutes photographers were crowding around. We had been on Japanese television news bulletins and in the media every day and we stuck out like a sore thumb in the streets, with everyone wanting to gather around or photograph the "miracle" baby.

When we left Japan a week later the press were at Osaka airport once again to see us board a plane to Honolulu. After just over 4,000 miles and eight and a half hours flying time we changed flights for a further five hour flight to San Francisco and that was followed by a flight to Miami. We stayed there for a week and on the plane from Miami back to London the pilot invited the family up on to the flight deck. He worked out that by the time we landed I had flown 29,425 miles, which worked out at more than 100 miles for every day of my life so far.

Now that may be remarkable but it is fairly easy stuff for a baby. You just lie around, cry and wait for food to be spooned into your mouth. But it was pretty tough for Mum and Dad. Anyone with a small baby will tell you how hard it is travelling. For Mum and Dad, who were hardly the most experienced travellers in the world, it was a pretty tough time and understandably affected their ability to smile on demand for the media.

The Florida part of the trip was hosted by the National Enquirer newspaper. I got a slight Florida tan, but more importantly by the time we returned home I had four more teeth. Before we left the UK I had two bottom teeth, two appeared in Japan and another two in America.

Mum told the Daily Mail on our return to the UK: "It's amazing the effect she has on people. Everybody we meet wants to take her home with them. She has become a very good air traveller - better than the rest of us."

While in Florida we had a two-day trip to Disneyland, where even the amazing Walt Disney Corporation were pleased to be associated with me and I was pictured in many newspapers wearing a Mickey Mouse Club hat and beaming away.

We had a little bit of downtime between the interviews with Dad cooking a barbecue for the family on a Florida beach.

Dad had used up his annual leave going to Japan. Mum and Dad had always wanted to see Scotland and with Grace now a firm friend they had an open invitation to head North. But our travels meant that Dad only had one week left of his annual leave, even though it was only March.

With the plans for the book to be published later in 1979 there were tough decisions to be made about the future.

Enough money had poured in to Chandlewise from the various media deals done around the world for Mum and Dad to feel confident about moving out of the little terraced house in Hassell Drive into something a bit bigger. They found a modest three-bedroomed house in the suburbs of Bristol.

Whitchurch was once a village on the main road between Bristol and the Somerset city of Wells. During the early part of the 20th century flat land to the South of Bristol had been developed into a mixture of Council housing estates and private homes. Building went right up to the base of the massive Dundry Hill, which towers like a green back-drop to South Bristol.

The estates of Knowle West, Hartcliffe, Highridge and Withywood had been developed as homes for salt-of-the-earth Bristol families. Many of them worked at the Wills Tobacco Factory, which first had been in Bedminster but had then been relocated to a new site near Hartcliffe.

What we called Whitchurch was the huge extension of the original village stretching towards the factory. The flat area had also once been the home of Bristol's Airport. When a new one was built outside of the city the old one was abandoned. For years local people learned to drive on its closed-down runways. The fields alongside the runway were a playground for all. One of the old airport hangers had been converted into a sports centre and a small athletics track. Mum and Dad loved the new area - the air was cleaner out of the city and there was more room.

They bought a house in Court Farm Road and that was where they stayed for the rest of their lives. It is the first house I remember and my first real memory is of Mum passing me over the back fence to a neighbour to try to hide me from a newspaper reporter that was outside the house trying to take my picture.

Mum couldn't have been happier with the house. There was a little garden at the back for me to play in, a rank of local shops just round the corner, good schools nearby and within walking distance an Asda supermarket, which within time both me and Mum would end up getting part-time jobs in.

Although they lived hundreds of miles apart Mum and Grace kept in touch regularly through telephone calls and letters. Mum and Dad were getting sick of the spotlight and were able to warn her about the dangers of co-operating with all the media requests and hype following the birth of Alastair.

As the year went on Dad took some unpaid time off so that the two families could be together in Scotland. It was strange that IVF had now brought two families at opposite ends of the country together as friends. It also meant that I had a little playmate in baby Alastair.

The book "Our Miracle Called Louise" came out in July with me chuckling away on the cover. Sue Freeman had made a good job of turning Mum and Dad's ramblings and matter-of-fact answers into a dramatic tale of a couple desperate for a baby, who eventually got their wish.

Mum and Dad thought it would stop the constant questions they had to answer - after all it would all be in the book and people could just look it up if they were that interested.

Of course that was completely wrong. The book was being published all over the world and that meant it had to be promoted and the media certainly weren't interested in talking to the real author Sue Freeman - they wanted to talk to the people whose name it had been written in, Mum and Dad, and also see how the "test-tube baby" had grown.

Paul Vincent agreed to a tour to promote the book so we were off on a promotional tour of the USA.

The publishers Paddington Press produced a schedule which saw us spending pretty much the whole of September 1979 travelling around the USA on what was called the "Our Miracle Called Louise - Fall '79" tour.

By "us" I mean me, Sharon, Mum and Dad, Paul Vincent and

assorted people from publishers or their US agents and counterparts. We flew out of London on a Trans World Airline Flight that saw us landing in Chicago on September 5. We didn't arrive back in the UK until September 30.

Although breaks were built in where the family could have days off and do a bit of sight-seeing it was a punishing schedule for parents with a 14 month old baby and a 17-year-old girl in tow.

I had started walking before I was a year old so like all toddlers a little bit harder for the group to control than it had been in Japan as I now had a tendency to get about.

Unlike rock stars and authors who might dream of such attention this was completely alien territory to Mum and Dad. They had never once wanted to tour the world and stay in endless hotels. They were happiest going shopping in Bristol and just bringing up their family.

The whole thing was made worse by the fact that the media in America often took the line of accusing Mum and Dad of "cashing in" on their baby. When they set off they thought the tour would be all about them telling everyone how wonderful IVF was and what a great difference it might be to the world.

In fact most interviewers were accusing them of going against the morals of the church, getting involved in some kind of Nazi-cloning programme, making money out of their precious child and all kinds of other nasty things. It seems few were interested in the story in the book - the story of a poor couple who just wanted a baby so much that they would do just about anything and how they had been helped by the work of Edwards and Steptoe and their team.

All of this was to dawn slowly on Mum and Dad as the tour went on. Tired after a long flight and coping with the time difference they were just happy to hop into the back of a limousine and be whisked to the Palmer House Hotel in Monroe Street, Chicago.

Mum with most of her luggage taken up with baby food and nappies could barely appreciate that they had been booked into a hotel that Charles Dickens and Oscar Wilde had also stayed in when they had been promoting their literature! Here was Dad with his tattoos and his HGV licence on leave from the railway in Bristol arriving at a swanky hotel as a "British author" just wanting to get his family settled and see if they had a pint of bitter in the bar - of course they didn't.

The hotel was delighted to welcome us as their latest "celebrity" guests. Apparently US Presidents and stars such as Judy Garland, Ella Fitzgerald, Harry Belafonte and Louis Armstrong had stayed in the suites reserved for us. Dad was more impressed to hear that Frank Sinatra had used our room!

There was little time to rest. The first media appointment was booked in for the next day - a half hour trip to the 19th floor of a tower block where someone called Dorothy Challob would meet the family and take us in to film The Today Show with a bloke called Phil Donahue.

Mum and Dad had never heard of the man, who became a legend in US television and who invented the talk show format that we are all familiar with these days. The first day was a brief taped interview for The Today Show and a chance for Phil Donahue to meet Mum and Dad and me and tell them what he was looking for the following day.

Donahue liked the way I said "Baba" when shown the picture of myself on the front of the book but otherwise he found it difficult having a toddler as the main subject for his show.

Friday September 7 we went to do the Phil Donahue Show. By that time it had been running for four years from Chicago and was just about the biggest show in America. Mum and Dad and me were to appear live and syndicated across the United States.

Phil Donahue explained that there would be a studio audience who would be invited to ask questions and give their views on what they thought about test-tube babies. The whole thing was being broadcast from the independent TV station WGN-TV.

Donahue introduced me as "a wonderful human being" and Mum carried me on to prime time US television wearing her best red dress with Dad by her side, parading through the studio audience.

Then while the people at home watched adverts for Shoprite Plus with its 57 cent chicken legs, Sipping Yoghurt, House of Pancakes and Lysol Cleaner Mum, Dad and me were seated behind a round table and microphones were put on Mum and Dad's clothing.

Well, I said seated but as Donahue introduced us with the words: "You imagine what this family has been through" I decided to crawl over the table take hold of Donahue's script and screw it up in my hand. Donahue had to grab me saying: "Hello Louise, I'm not David Frost!" to get a laugh.

Knowing from the meeting the day before the reaction it would get he held up the book to me and I grabbed it and said: "Baba" before setting off again to squirm across the table. A flustered Donahue could only say: "This is an active child." Mum grabbed me but that meant I was then gabbling baby talk loudly into the microphone and Donahue had to ask a technician to kill Mum's mic so that I didn't drown out the chat on his chat show. It wasn't going well as far as he was concerned.

Dad told how the media spotlight had affected the family initially and described the siege at Hassell Drive, saying "we locked ourselves away frightened to go anywhere" but then said that things were now much better. The serious discussion about press intrusion was interrupted by a toddler in a blue frilly dress shouting "Baba" - yes it was me again determined to make the most of a major talk show appearance.

Donahue forgot his question - or maybe he couldn't find it because I now had another piece of his script firmly in my grasp. Besides not many of the audience were actually listening to him anyway as I was now gripping the edge of the table and threatening to throw myself over the edge. The drama of a toddler plummeting off the table with a big wide grin on its face was far more entertaining than the chat.

Donahue eventually grabbed me and said: "I'm getting nowhere with this child" and Sharon, who had been summoned by a floor manager came and carried me out of shot and to the back of the studio to try to keep me quiet.

An expert Dr Pierre Soupart of the Vanderbilt University Medical centre in Nashville Tenessee, one of the USA's foremost experts in reproductive biology was then introduced and Mum and Dad were able to relax a little as he explained what IVF was and even brought a few pieces of equipment along to explain the medical procedure. Dad thought it was most amusing as the eminent scientist got bits of glassware out of boxes and showed Donahue how eggs were removed and implanted back into women with blocked fallopian tubes.

The early part of his expert contribution was interrupted by me shouting from the back of the studio. Donahue eventually had to say: "Baby Louise doesn't like me and doesn't like my show" before eventually Sharon was able to keep me quiet by shoving a bottle of juice into my mouth.

During the next commercial break the studio decided that the best thing to do might be to let me run around amongst the studio audience. But of course it would be hard for the camera to keep track of me so they tied a pink balloon to my wrist so that I could be tracked as I wandered around. Some local newspaper cameramen were invited to take pictures of me and as we came back on air I could be seen standing steadfastly with my back to them with the balloon on my wrist.

Donahue said: "You'll never be a star if you don't face the camera Louise." The discussion moved on to whether Mum and Dad would go through the process again and they said they definitely would and Dr Soupart said that he believed that IVF - which by now successfully brought three children into the world would be commonplace within 10 years.

The studio audience were invited to have a say and one woman expressed fears that the technique could be used to allow two women to have a child between them. Other moral questions are asked and a man wondered whether thoroughbred horses could be bred in this way, before Dr Soupart informed him they already are.

People asked what if the technique got into the hands of a "Hitler type personality" and another said that the circumstances of my birth "boggles the mind". At one point the adults got so deep in discussion they forgot all about the toddler until there was an anguished cry as I plummeted over a step at the back of the studio and Donahue rushed to pick me up.

Just as they did in every media interview Mum and Dad told everyone that they would inform me of the unusual nature of my birth as soon as I was old enough to understand. They also said they intended for me to have as normal as possible a childhood.

Dr Soupart pointed out how IVF could be used to determine whether a baby was going to be healthy and - if necessary - terminated. The mother of a 24-year-old boy with cerebral palsy told how she wouldn't have wanted that to happen as that would have meant she would have missed out on knowing her wonderful son.

So, with me causing chaos, our first major appearance on US television was over. Afterwards other press people were able to question Mum and Dad with the same questions again before we were taken back to the hotel.

Later Donahue told a reporter: "I cannot bring any real moral indignation to this thing. I think they're entitled to this, really. This is not the Carnival Midway. I honestly was not offended. I saw two people who, I think, love their baby. The issue to me is not whether they want to sell a book - it is whether they love their child."

The next morning we all had to be up early because our flight out of Chicago was at 7.25am heading for Toronto, Canada. At 10am Don Bradstreet, President of the Random House publishers in Canada met our party as we arrived at Toronto Airport and we were whisked to the Castle Harbor Hilton.

Just two years earlier the Rolling Stones were staying at this same hotel when a drug bust by the Mounties had made the news all over the world. It was mid-morning before we got there after a hectic couple of days. The schedule said we had a free day for sight-seeing but Mum and Dad just wanted to rest. From our bedroom there was a view of the CN Tower.

The next day was Sunday so to make life a little easier the publishers had arranged for a reporter and a photographer from the Toronto Star to come to the hotel for the interview. After another round of the usual questions Dan Bradstreet took the whole family to lunch then to Niagara Falls for a bit of sight-seeing.

The relentless schedule continued the next day starting at 8.30am with a taped interview for Canada AM television; then another TV appearance at 10am on City Pulse News being interviewed by Ly Macintern. This was followed immediately at 11.30am with an interview with Toronto Sun journalist Cathy Brun back at the hotel. Then a quick lunch and we were paraded in front of Canadian Press for an interview with Judy Crighton, immediately followed by an interview with the Globe and Mail. Just to round off the day there was an interview with Global TV News at 4.15pm and CBC-TV at 5.30pm.

Mum and Dad slumped exhausted into bed that night but it was another early start the next day as we all had to be at the airport for a 7.30am take-off to Detroit where we landed at 8.15am.

There we were all checked into another high rise hotel - the Pontchartrain on Washington Boulevard. But there was barely time to put down the bags.

A car was already waiting outside to take us to WDIV-TV in West Lafayette for a recorded interview with Cheryl Friske on WWJ Radio, an interview with Nikki McCrowder of Detroit Free Press then a live half-hour television appearance with Deena Pearlman on WDVI-TV. The publishers then obligingly agreed to an extra bit of filming with the television channel that night at 7pm.

By now Mum and Dad were just about fed up with being asked the same questions over and over again. All questions that were answered in the book, which they had co-operated with precisely because they didn't want to go through this sort of interview. So it is no wonder that their interviews were getting worse and worse.

Cheryl Friske described her encounter with Mum and Dad: "Two of the most common ordinary people I've ever met. After a year of dealing with reporters, I at least expected her to be able to talk!"

Next morning was a very early call - why? You've guessed it the family from Britain had to be bright-eyed and bushy-tailed on AM Detroit from 6.45am through to 8am. Now looking distinctly sullen and fed up Mum and Dad were quizzed by reporter Georgette Turken. A car was waiting outside to get them to Detroit airport as there was a flight at 9am landing at Los Angeles at 10.21am.

Unpacking their bags at the Beverley Rodeo Hotel in North Rodeo Drive, Beverley Hills Mum and Dad hardly had time to reflect on the fact that here they were in the heart of celebrity-land. They had a fed-up teenager and a tired toddler on their hands.

Their latest host told them that they could have a few hours to rest before a limousine would pick them up at 5.30pm for the taping of the Mike Douglas Show. The fact this was a major television programme - famous for being interrupted in 1963 with first reports of the assassination of John F Kennedy were coming in, was totally lost on Mum and Dad and me... to us it was just another person asking the same old questions about the birth, the newspaper reactions, whether I had anything wrong with me and what they planned to do in the future.

A few hours back at the hotel and next day we were taken to Prospect Avenue for a 90-minute appearance on AM Los Angeles. There was just enough time to grab a bit of lunch then it was off to the airport for another flight - just over two hours on a plane from Los Angeles to Portland, Oregon. It was well into the late evening and way past the bedtime of a 14 month old baby before the family checked into the magnificent grand lobby of the Benson Hotel. Mum couldn't care less about the stunning architecture or the fact that US Presidents had stayed here before her. She just wanted to get the baby bathed and fed and in bed. Not least because Jonathan Milkes, the book salesman for the area, who had met us at the airport, had just told us that he would be back early the next day as we were due on AM Northwest at 8.30am; that we had to do a book signing at JK Gill bookshop from Noon to 2pm after that and that we would be taping a section for Sunday Morning on KATU TV at 8pm that night.

By now journalists were finding the family from the UK were acting distinctly surly. In truth Mum and Dad and Sharon had little idea about how to behave in the weird circumstances they were finding themselves. There were times that they felt their baby was being treated a bit like a freak show and just being paraded and they didn't like it.

Just how many times can you say: "We want her to grow up to be as normal as possible" without sounding bored at hearing the same question again? Just how many times did they want to know from Mum whether the procedure was painful?: "No, I didn't feel a thing." Just how often did they want to know what Mum and Dad thought of Edwards and Steptoe? "We are so grateful - they have brought us joy".

To be fair Dad probably enjoyed it a bit more than Mum. He had more of an out-going personality and, after all, if there was a dirty nappy to be changed seconds before going on air, a feeding time to remember or the baby's hair to comb, well that was women's work and Mum had to do it!

But really neither of them were entertainers or actors and that was what the media wanted them to be. Why should a lorry driver from Bristol and his wife, who had worked in an underwear factory, suddenly make interesting television just because they had a baby? They simply grunted answers to the questions, which were getting boring in their repetition while I smiled and gurgled and toddled. Soon the word went around the USA media: "They are nice people, but bad guests." The tour was getting boring for both sides!

Margie Boule, who interviewed Mum for AM Northwest in Portland said: "I feel sorry for her. She's just so painfully shy. I'm sure she's just doing this because she feels they couldn't support the baby without this tour."

Saturday September 15 waking up at the Benson Hotel, Portland the family packed the bags once again and headed for the 10.25am flight to San Francisco - arriving at mid-day. It was a great day because recognising that they just couldn't take any more the family were given a couple of days off. Well by the time they had checked into the Travel Lodge at the Wharf Hotel it was only a day and a half but it was very welcome.

There was a bit of sight-seeing in San Francisco but Mum was also able to stock up on baby things and enjoy a weekend without the press firing questions every minute of every day. It was also a relief to know that this was a hotel that would be home for three nights - so the bags could be properly unpacked and there were no aeroplane flights.

The constant changes in air pressure on the flights had played havoc with Mum's ears, which had been quite painful on some descents and she was pleased to have a few days to get them back to normal.

Monday our only appearance was on This Morning with KPIX, who laughingly billed the appearance by the family as "live and exclusive" before asking all the same questions as everyone else.

The next day we flew from San Francisco to Houston, Texas, where there were reporters waiting to snatch pictures at the airport before we checked in to the Ramada Inn, South West Freeway. Despite the fact that we had just been on a flight for over five hours there was only time to drop the bags and then go to a live TV interview at KPRC TV in a programme called Scene At Five.

The next day was equally hectic. First thing in the morning it was an interview with Don Nelson at KTRK TV Live for the Good Morning Houston show. The cracks were beginning to show with Dad and Don Nelson said afterwards of him: "The guy's just living hand to mouth. There's a lot of pressure on him to make sure the kid lives right."

Straight after that interview we were whisked across town to another studio to be interviewed by MaryJan Vandivier for a programme called Calendar.

Mum and Dad were fed up and making their views known to those who had arranged the tour. There had been one bit of the trip to the

USA that Dad had been really been looking forward to and that was going to Memphis. Dad was a huge Elvis Presley fan. The death of the "King of Rock and Roll" in August 1977 had been a sad day for him, as it was for all Elvis fans across the world.

He had seen film of Graceland but as a lorry driver in Bristol he never dreamed he would ever get a chance to go to Memphis and see the house himself. So when the tour was being arranged he asked if it was possible.

A planned appearance signing books at Foley's Department Store in Houston was cancelled and the family flew to Memphis a day early. Checked into the Hyatt Regency Hotel on Ridge Lake Boulevard we had three days with no press interviews and no television or radio appearances.

It was a time to recharge the batteries. Mum found a nice restaurant called the Knickerbocker on Poplar, where the family were able to get a taste of the USA at last away from hotels and the spotlight. Of course we had been on TV so much that we were recognised a few times and people wanted to come up and peer at the "test-tube baby" but mostly it was family time and for Dad the ultimate treat - a visit to see the grave of Elvis Presley and the gates of Graceland and a chance to buy some Elvis souvenirs.

It was a slightly happier family that boarded the 5.35pm Braniff airline flight from Memphis to Washington DC on Saturday September 22. After a three hour flight and another limousine ride we were checked into the Mayflower Hotel on Connecticut Avenue.

The hotel boasts that it is Washington's "second best address" meaning it is second only to the White House and a whole parade of American President's had been through its doors over the years. It was the last week of our American tour and Mum at last felt that she was close to boarding the one plane she wanted to get on - the one that would take her back home to England and her own bed!

Monday saw an interview on the phone live into WBBG in Cleveland, Ohio, which had come in as a late request. That evening

Mum and Dad were broadcast live lying on their hotel bed on the telephone in an interview with Carole Hemingway for her show on KABC Radio.

The next morning Tony Kornheiser of the Washington Post met us in our hotel room. His account in the paper told of me playing with Mum's feet and he quoted Dad talking in his Bristol accent as saying: "I think people had the impression we'd lock 'er away and say -"Do Not Touch", But what's the big deal? We've never 'id 'er away. We came to America to show 'er off to people, to show 'em she's normal."

He said of me: "Baby Louise was in motion. Walking, running, climbing, reaching, grabbing, falling, bouncing. Baby Louise was unbreakable. And unstoppable. The book was laying on the bed in the hotel room and as soon as Baby Louise saw it, she went for it. She picked it up, turned it upside down then right side up and stared at the colour photograph of the baby on the cover.

"Who's that?" her father asked. "Who you lookin' at Lou-lu?" her mother asked.

Baby Louise was looking at baby Louise smiling at her from the cover of "Our Miracle Called Louise" by Lesley and John Brown. Baby Louise gurgles. Baby Louise pointed. Baby Louise said "Baba". Then baby Louise tossed the book to the floor. Just another pretty face."

Tony Kornheiser painted the first real picture of Mum and Dad in America, mentioned how they had been nicking soap from the hotels to take home; how much they hated the term "test-tube baby" and how worried Mum was that they wouldn't be good parents.

He chatted to Sharon and got her view on it and he demonstrated how ordinary Mum and Dad were by pointing out that Dad had no idea what the word "semen" meant when he had to have his sperm tested and that Mum had been slow on the uptake in realising that human life had never been produced "in vitro" before when she agreed to the procedure.

Tony Kornheiser left and the family were taken to WTTG TV to do a live piece on the programme Panorama. Before leaving the studio there was a newspaper interview with Jo Clendenron of the Baltimore Herald. Then we were driven to Baltimore for a night at the Cross Keys Inn, Falls Road.

After breakfast Terry Rubinstein of the Baltimore Sun came to the hotel with the usual clutch of questions before another limousine ride to appear on Two's Company, a live TV show at WMAR TV. That afternoon we flew to New York and, yet another hotel: the Salisbury on 57th Street.

The press were getting bored of the matter-of-fact British family by now so only one interview - on AM New York the next day before we boarded a shuttle flight from LaGuardia Airport to Boston and our final two nights in the USA at the Marriott Inn, Commonwealth Avenue.

Friday September 28 saw us appear on Good Day! on WCVB TV and do an interview with the Boston Globe. Saturday was supposed to be a day of sight-seeing but Mum couldn't wait for 9pm that evening to come around when our flight lifted off taking us back to London and finally home to Bristol.

As soon as they got home and through the doors at Court Farm Road Mum and Dad pledged that they had to get back to normal. It was obvious the media spotlight wasn't for them.

In one of his last interviews in America Dad had said: "Let me tell you - no more books, no more tours. This is it. Now we're going back home and be normal again. Mr. and Mrs. Johnny Brown and family, I drive me truck. I enjoy me work."

The world tour of 1979 had taken its toll.

Chapter 7

MOVIE PLANS
AND IVF MOVES ON

A lthough we were all back home safely in Bristol it seemed that the USA had followed us home. The journalists may not have been terribly impressed with the interviews Mum and Dad gave but the public bought the book and once again letters started arriving every day from all corners of the States.

Within weeks of being back at Court Farm Road there was interest in making a Hollywood movie about my birth. CBS and Universal Television announced that they were planning the movie, which would probably go straight on to television.

World famous producer Carl Foreman CBE said that he was planning to turn the book into a movie that would "focus on the human drama and real life love story that brought about the scientific breakthrough."

Carl Foreman was living in the UK at the time and had an office in Jermyn Street, London. Originally from Chicago he had come to the UK after being blacklisted in Hollywood during the 1950s events that became known as the McCarthy "witch hunts".

He had written the screenplay for *High Noon* and in 1951 had been summoned to appear before the House Committee of Un-American

Activities. He had admitted that 10 years before he had been a member of the Communist Party but refused to name others so was effectively banned from working in the USA.

High Noon came out in 1952 to critical acclaim but as a blacklisted writer Foreman found life very difficult in 1950s America. He had been one of the top writers in Hollywood but had to move to the UK where he continued to write.

Like many others banned from working in Hollywood he got around the blacklisting by using pseudonyms and while in England he wrote *The Bridge on the River Kwai* which won an Oscar without him getting the credit until years later. He also wrote *The Guns of Navarone* and *Born Free* and got his CBE in 1970 for services to the British Film Industry.

Carl Foreman was honoured by the British Film Industry. A BAFTA for Most Promising Newcomer was named after him from 1998 to 2008. Well, in October 1979 after our successful tour of the USA his secretary Eileen Wood made arrangements for him to come to the little three-bedroom house in Whitchurch, Bristol and meet Mum and Dad, me and Sharon.

Most of the arrangements were made through Paul Vincent, who saw the Hollywood film as another earner for Chandlewise. Carl Foreman and his wife Estelle travelled by train from London to Temple Meads, Bristol on November 8 then got a taxi to Whitchurch arriving at 4pm for a chat and a cup of tea. They got on well with Mum and Dad.

They had got hold of video tapes of television shows we had been on during the trip across the USA and promised to make copies. True to their word the tapes - copied from the American format into something playable in the UK arrived just in time for Christmas 1979. Carl Foreman said copying the tapes had been "a long, expensive and difficult process" and he couldn't get the sound right on some of them. Interestingly his note to Mum said:"I am enclosing the original tapes, as well as the new one, in the hope that perhaps some day, when all recording machines are compatible, you may be able to run them as well," which showed he was quite forward thinking.

By the time that Christmas parcel arrived the script for the film was already under-way, being written by Gillian Freeman. But it was a full nine months before a big parcel arrived with the script in a yellow "Universal Studios" cover with a note from Mr. Foreman.

He said: "Sorry it has taken so long, but there have been so many problems in Hollywood lately, some of which you may have read about, such as the actors' strike and the musicians strike etc."

He warned Mum and Dad that they might find it a bit strange reading a film script about themselves. He said: "There are some things that cannot be shown exactly as they took place for one reason or another and what we have tried to do is to be faithful to the spirit of your book and to the miracle that you two and Louise and the two doctors were part of.

"One or other of you may say "But that isn't the real me". Well, the answer to that is that no one really knows who we really are, and in making a film one tries to show a character or person that people will like and be concerned about. Also, you will find certain things left out and certain things that didn't happen in exactly the way they are shown or at exactly the same time, but here again I remind you that our objective is to make a film and not a book or a biography, and most importantly a film that will amuse and inspire and entertain and touch people all over the world."

The plan was to look for locations around Bristol to do some of the filming. Mum and Dad looked through the script and did find some bits embarrassing - especially the bedroom scenes. Of course Patrick Steptoe and Bob Edwards were also portrayed in the script and Paul Vincent got involved in ensuring that they were happy with the script. That proved really difficult because they wanted to make sure that IVF was properly portrayed and there was a lot of to-ing and fro-ing between the legal teams before Paul Vincent was able to tell Carl Foreman that they were happy with the whole idea of a film.

That legal wrangle and the fact that Steptoe and Edwards were very busy trying to establish their first clinic meant the project went into 1981. Carl Foreman was spending a lot of time, effort and money flying backwards and forwards to Hollywood. By April a third revised screenplay had been produced by Gillian Freeman and Jon Elliott, who had been brought in.

In June 1981 Carl Foreman and his wife flew to the UK as his wife's mother was seriously ill with emphysema and he took the opportunity to tell Mum and Dad the latest.

He said: "We had been very happy because we had finally gotten everything straightened out with Mr. Steptoe and Dr. Edwards, but just as this was done we had a series of strikes in Hollywood, the most important one being the writers' strike which is on now, and the fact that the directors may go on strike in a week or two.

"Under these circumstances our plans and hopes to begin actual production this August are now considerably up in the air. I have no idea when or if the position will improve, although I hope and believe that things will work out and that the whole situation will be straightened out some time this summer. If that is the case then, hopefully we will be able to make the film this year after all, and at long last."

The actress Lynn Redgrave, a member of the famous British acting dynasty was lined up to play the part of Mum. She had been making quite a name for herself on Broadway and in the movies. Dad was to be played by Ian McShane, who was famous for his role on British television as Lovejoy. He later went on to gain fame in the USA in the series Deadwood.

In fact production 85557 "A Miracle Called Louise" never got beyond script form. By October 1981 Universal Studios had pulled the funding on it and Carl Foreman was looking for alternative finance. Universal Studios had paid some money in option fees and the amount paid to Chandlewise was just over £3,000, although once again some newspapers reported that Mum and Dad had made a fortune out of a movie deal.

Another result of our trip to America was a number of "fan letters" I received. One parcel arrived from a girl called Christine Santiago from Bronxville just north of New York City. It was addressed simply to Louise Brown, Test-tube Baby, Bristol, England. It found us.

Inside was a blue and white dress and a card with flowers on. The neat handwriting started: "Dear Louise, I know that you may not be able to read this letter, so I'm hoping that your Mom will read it to you. I know you don't know me but I am one of your many admirers who thinks you are the cutest, most adorable baby in the world."

Christina Santiago was just 16 years old and had the idea to write because she was doing a school health class assignment and had decided to write about IVF as it had been in the news. She had been to England when she was nine years old and loved everything about England - so she had another agenda in trying to reach out to someone on the other side of the Atlantic.

Her Mum had helped her pick out the blue and white dress and she had decided to send it to me for my second birthday. She ended the letter: "Your American Friend". The parcel had bounced back to them once after being addressed to the American publishers of the book, but the family had persevered even though they didn't know our address.

The dress fitted perfectly and Mum loved it. She took a picture of me wearing it on the beach at Weston-super-Mare and sent the photo back to Christina at her home in Kraft Avenue, Bronxville.

Christina couldn't have been happier to get her own picture of me wearing the dress she had sent and wrote back a letter of thanks. That was the beginning of a friendship that was to last many years. Christina still has the photo Mum sent in a scrapbook and we keep in touch and have met up many times over the years.

Christina's was one of dozens of letters from America that arrived following the publication of the book and the promotional tour of the States. Again they were mostly from women who had problems conceiving a child and who wanted to ask questions of Mum - the vast majority of them wanted to know more about IVF and how they could get in touch with Patrick Steptoe and Bob Edwards.

What Mum didn't know at that time is that my birth had already sparked off events in the USA that meant an IVF programme was being developed.

Howard Jones and his wife Georgeanna from Baltimore, USA already had a growing reputation for their work in fertility. Georgeanna, while at Johns Hopkins University had developed many of the first reliable pregnancy testing kits.

They had met Bob Edwards many years before and had exchanged notes and encouraged each other over the years. Dr Howard had spoken up in support of Bob Edwards when biomedical ethics were discussed in the USA.

On the day I was born Howard and Georgeanna were moving to Norfolk, Virginia after accepting posts at the Eastern Virginia Medical School. A woman reporter arrived at their house and the obliging Dr Howard Jones sat on some packing cases fascinated to hear that Bob Edwards and Patrick Steptoe had been successful in creating an IVF baby. He was questioned for his opinion as an expert.

Just about the last question the reporter asked was: "Do you think it would be possible to create test-tube babies in America?" Dr Jones replied that there was no reason why the work of Steptoe and Edwards couldn't be replicated in the USA. The reporter asked "What is the biggest barrier to creating a test-tube baby?" and Jones replied: "Money. It would cost quite a bit to get set up."

A report duly appeared in the local paper the next day and of course the reporter said that money was the only obstacle to an IVF programme being set up in Virginia. That day a rich former patient of Georgeanna rang up and said she had read the newspaper report and wanted to donate money. A meeting was held later that day - amid the packing cases of the Jones' new home and the idea for the Jones Institute for Reproductive Medicine was born.

They faced a lot of initial opposition but eventually set up in March 1980 and were inundated with requests from women wanting treatment - Mum could have given them a whole batch of names from her own postbag.

It took some time before they perfected their technique and they worked on methods involving strong fertility drugs to encourage women to produce more eggs. Around a year after the clinic opened a lady called Judy Carr got pregnant through their methods and her daughter Elizabeth Jordan Carr became America's first test-tube baby born on December 28, 1981. She was the 15th baby to be born in the world through IVF - because Steptoe and Edwards had been busy with their own venture!

Steptoe had reached the statutory retirement age pretty much as I was born and that meant he could no longer work for the NHS. The reluctance of Steptoe and Edwards to bow to the pressure of publishing their methods early meant they had come in for some criticism. But both were determined to continue to develop the work of IVF.

In 1980 they opened Bourn Hall Clinic. Set in 22 acres of land in Cambridgeshire it had originally been a Jacobean House with a history dating back to 1602. Other parts of the house had been built in 1817. It was to become the world's first IVF centre.

As well as the two amazing men Bourn Hall would not have happened without the work of Jean Purdy, the woman who had first seen the cells dividing in the petri dish that later turned into me. From all accounts she was an amazing woman. She worked hard towards turning the old Jacobean manor house into a working clinic with a laboratory where IVF could be carried out and did a lot of the work in smoothing things between the two very different personalities of Steptoe and Edwards. My Mum always said she was an unsung hero and that without her, IVF babies may never have been a reality.

Bourn Hall became a place that I was to visit many times over the years - and still do. Mum and Dad saw how important it was to the two founders. Just as predicted by the experts when I was born - I was no longer a novelty. As each of the other IVF babies were born it was becoming more and more commonplace but still the press could not get enough of the story and Mum and Dad's pledge to keep a low profile proved difficult to keep.

The fifth test-tube baby was named Natalie Curtis and her parents agreed to take part in a documentary and there were articles in the paper. Mum had never heard the name Natalie before - but she liked it. Natalie's Mum was surprised to get a call from my Mum, who said she liked the name Natalie and would she mind if she named a future daughter of hers by the same name.

By the time I was two Mum was thinking about whether she dare ask Edwards and Steptoe again if she could try for a little sister or brother for me. There were scary headlines in the newspapers about Bourn Hall, such as: "Hidden world of the test-tube baby farm" where reporters went under cover trying to expose some scandal about the place.

But all they found was Bob Edwards nailing down the carpets and Patrick Steptoe carrying beds in for patients. There was nothing but praise from those who went there in the hope of conceiving a baby. The ethics of Edwards and Steptoe were constantly being questioned by the British Medical Association.

Mum wanted another baby but at the same time was reading items in the press as outraged anti-abortionists accused Edwards of "playing God" and called for a ban on "experiments" on embryos. There were even calls for the doctors to be arrested. In almost every story it would mention me and keep the name "Louise Brown" in the headlines. Pictures of me doing almost anything were in demand from the Fleet Street editors and journalists all over the world.

Hardly a day went by without a journalist coming to the door or writing or ringing with a question for Mum and Dad. Usually they were questions that they had no idea how to answer or were hardly qualified to have an opinion on.

"What did they think of the idea of cloning?" "What did they think of the fact that people were paying over £1,000 to have IVF treatment?" "What were their views on embryos being frozen for future use?" "How far did they think people should go in experimenting on human embryos?"

Then there were the personal questions: "Has Louise got any health problems?" "How do you think she will cope with the fame?" "Has being the parents of the first test-tube baby put a strain on your marriage?" "Is it true you have argued with the neighbours?"

The family got more and more fed up and less and less co-operative. There were still some promotional events for the book arranged. We went to BBC Television Centre in Shepherd's Bush, London to spend an afternoon recording for the programme "All About Books With Russell Harty" and the local television stations and newspapers were still knocking on the door every week or so.

In a conversation with Patrick Steptoe, Mum mentioned that she would like another baby. She was so modest that she felt that she didn't deserve to have another as she had been so fortunate to have found the two doctors and to have had a successful pregnancy. She felt that other women who wanted babies should get priority.

But Patrick Steptoe said there was no reason why she shouldn't have another baby and welcomed her to Bourn Hall for another treatment. The newspapers were full of stories of women who had spent a lot of money on IVF - some taking out bank loans - and then not conceiving. People were beginning to question whether there might be a scam involved with money being taken off women who had no chance of conceiving.

For Mum the treatment worked again - first time. She was pregnant again. Mum and Dad paid for the treatment at Bourn Hall and were treated exactly the same as any other patient - although I suspect there was always a special interest from Edwards and Steptoe on the progress of the pregnancy - after all this was the woman who showed with the momentous occasion of the birth of the first IVF baby that their work over the years could be successful.

The IVF treatments cost Mum and Dad £2,000, including travelling expenses to and from Bourn Hall in Cambridgeshire from our home in Bristol. By this time IVF pregnancies were not under any special scrutiny so Mum attended the hospital in Bristol and was booked in to have a cesarean operation to deliver the baby on June 30, 1982.

But two weeks early she was rushed in to Bristol Maternity Hospital, so on June 14 1982 my baby sister popped into the world weighing in at 5lb 15 oz. Of course Mum called her Natalie Jane and she has been in a hurry to do things ever since. I had someone to play and fight and argue with for the rest of my life and Mum had another precious child.

Of course Natalie's birth meant Mum was now the first woman in the world to have two IVF pregnancies. It made the news and Dad told reporters the next day: "I think I've had enough now. We are going to call it a day. I am getting on a bit and we will give the young people a chance."

Years later Mum was to say: "Natalie was really special to me. I always felt I had to share Louise with the whole world because she was the first through IVF. Natalie was all mine, just for me and nobody else."

Natalie was the 40th IVF baby to be born in the world - thanks to the sterling work of Edwards and Steptoe and the other clinics beginning to spring up around the world.

That September I was due to leave the playgroup I had been attending at St Augustine's Church, just around the corner from where I lived and go to primary school for the first time. Mum and Dad feared that I might get some odd treatment so she went to see the head teacher at Wansdyke School to explain about the constant press interest and to ensure that the teachers looked out for reporters and photographers.

Unlike today there was no security at schools and anyone could wander in and get to the classroom in which I was being taught.

Mum was also worried that other children might be told about me by their parents and might say cruel things to me. Generally, in Whitchurch people took our weird celebrity in their stride but from time to time someone would say something annoying.

Once a nearby newsagent said to a customer when Mum came in: "Here she is. The woman who has made a fortune out of having those babies." Of course people believed all the rubbish they read in the papers but after a while it was clear from Mum and Dad's lifestyle that they didn't have more than anyone else in the area - yes they had made some money out of selling their story but they had started from having nothing in the first place. Chandlewise had also been paying out on those hotels and legal bills.

Anyway, Mum thought it was best to make her first attempt at explaining to me about my birth. Agony Aunt Marje Proops had written a piece in the Daily Mirror saying how I should be told that I grew in Mummy's tummy just like everyone else but I needed a bit of help from doctors to get there.

Mum pretty much followed that advice, which she cut out of the newspaper. She sat me down and showed me the Central Office of Information film of my birth. I don't know what any four-year-old would make of a cesarean section! I certainly thought it looked pretty gruesome. It's hard enough for a young kid to understand where babies come from, but to then be told that it was a bit different with you only adds to the complication.

I wasn't really bothered by it all. I understood something different had happened around the time of my birth and that was why whenever I had a birthday or Christmas I appeared in the paper. That was about it. I can't say I understood it all, but I took it all in my stride and it didn't really affect me.

One of my earliest memories is walking to school holding my Mum's hand aged four. Natalie was in the pram just months old and as we walked towards the school a press photographer appeared ahead. Mum turned around and walked back towards the house and a reporter was heading towards us from the opposite direction. Mum dashed back into the house and got a neighbour called Val Kelly, whose husband was a policeman, to lift me over the fence and she took me to school in her car.

Most of my childhood involved tussling with Natalie. There is a bit of video of me wiping her nose when she was a small baby and it looks like I'm trying to tear her nose off. That was the kind of relationship we had. Always battling with each other.

We played together in the garden and we were quite close but it usually ended in a fight. I don't know why, maybe because there was so much happening around me, but I don't have many memories of my early years.

My Nanny Jean and Grandad Roy (Mum's stepfather) used to come around every Friday and spend time with us girls. Every Friday Mum would serve up a chicken wing with chicken seasoning along with diced salad with egg and cheese in it with vinegar in a bowl all in little cubes. Me and Natalie used to love that Friday night treat with our grandparents. I've tried many times to make that salad but never been able to make it taste the way Mum did - I could eat it now!

After the meal Nanny and Grandad would always give us a bag of sherbet pips each to have after the meal as our treat for a Friday night. Nanny Jean would sometimes take us to Bristol Zoo to see the exotic animals, which in those days included gorillas, white tigers, an elephant called Wendy and polar bears.

Every year Nanny Jean would make me and Natalie birthday cakes with rosewater, which we both thought were lush! Often I would be sent a birthday cake by some media organisation or somebody who was after publicity - Mum would accept them gracefully but give them to the Bristol Children's Hospital - Nanny Jean's was the real birthday cake for me!

Nanny Jean would also take us to St Ursula's School fete on a Saturday and me and Natalie both won goldfish and carried them home proudly in a polythene bag. We would spend time with her on Durdham Downs in Bristol, a vast green area and she would tell us tales about the "Seven sisters" - seven trees that stood tall - as we ran around the open space. Sometimes Grandad Roy, my Mum's step-father, would be with us.

We often visited my Mum's brother Uncle David and his wife Auntie Jill who lived in Kingswood, Bristol and see our cousins Kevin and Andrew, eating cheese and ham rolls to our heart's content. We went on family holidays to Swanage and Cornwall with them and I have fond memories of those seaside trips. Despite the strange beginnings and dire warnings from the media I had a pretty regular childhood for someone growing up in the South West of England.

Auntie Jill and Sharon seemed to have the same taste and on several occasions bought identical presents for me for birthdays or at Christmas, which became a bit of a family joke.

Mum needn't have worried about the children at school. I had a very normal childhood and the "test-tube baby" thing hardly got a mention, unless, of course I had made an appearance on television or in the newspapers. The children I grew up with went all through school with me and few of them even mentioned it.

I can remember one incident when someone came up to me in the playground and asked: "How did you fit in that test-tube as you are so fat" but I think people would use any bit of banter to have a go at someone if they wanted to and it was just the normal playground remarks that you get.

From being a celebrity baby, known all over the world, I became an anonymous schoolkid called Louise that just played in the playground with everyone else and joined in lessons.

But every now and then something odd would happen. Like when I was five years old and the Amercian newspaper the National Enquirer decided to do a colour picture special on me and Natalie at Christmas. In all their photos I was grinning away with a huge gap where my teeth should be as I had lost my baby teeth and my others hadn't arrived. They brought a rocking horse for me and took pictures of me with a gap-toothed grin riding the horse while holding on to Natalie in a ghastly green all-in-one baby suit.

Then Natalie opened her present from the National Enquirer - a massive cuddly stuffed giraffe. The paper reported that both of us "whooping with joy" and "shrieking with delight" at the gifts from America.

The paper measured and weighed us reporting that I was 3 feet 10 inches tall and weighed 55 pounds and that Natalie was 2 feet six inches tall and weighed 21 pounds. I don't suppose any other kids in South Bristol had their measurements reported to people on the other side of the world or received gifts that they were told were from "the people of America".

Chapter 8

SCHOOL DAYS

Growing up in South Bristol in the 1980s was pretty unremarkable for me. The people in that area take everything in their stride and, although everyone knew I was "the test-tube baby" it was rarely mentioned and, thankfully, there was no difference in the way I was treated to everyone else.

When I was just two years old there had been riots in St Paul's, Bristol, which showed there was underlying unrest in the city. The riots had involved a lot of the West Indian community in the areas where Mum and Dad had originally lived when they first moved in together.

The south of the city had just as many social problems but the working class, mostly white, neighbourhoods didn't show signs of civil unrest until I was a teenager. Many people were getting used to being home owners and shareholders. Many had bought their council house or small private house, like Mum and Dad, and they were becoming shareholders in British Gas, BT, banks and building societies. Because house prices were rising people felt they were making more money than ever.

There was the rise of "white van man" and his home was often in South Bristol. So-called because they often drove a white van with the tools of their trade these men were plumbers, alarm engineers, bricklayers and running their own businesses - sometimes working for cash and doing jobs on the side. They were the sort of people Dad mixed with when he went to the pub and he always had a mate that could come around and fix something or help out if the family needed anything.

Outside of school I spent most of my time watching TV with Natalie with programmes like Blue Peter coming from those same studios that I had appeared in as a toddler. When we weren't watching television we were in the garden playing on a swing.

At Wansdyke School nobody took any special interest in me. I went through the school years with the same group of friends who all played around the streets of South Bristol and in the open spaces of Whitchurch.

In 1983 we went to America again - this time with Natalie. Mum and Dad arranged to meet Christina Santiago and her family in New York. Her Mum and Dad took my Mum and Dad to the top of the World Trade Center building for a meal. I had just learned to write my name properly in school so I was delighted when Christina asked me to sign a copy of "Our Miracle Called Louise". She was the first person in the world to get an autograph and signed book from me! The two families got on well and it cemented my friendship with Christina.

This time around we weren't publicising the book but I was still the attraction for the media as the visit was used to announce some major steps forward in IVF. The whole trip was financed by the medical community. At Northridge Hospital Medical Center in the Northridge district of California I was paraded at a press conference.

The hospital boasted the only test in America that could detect in a brief time the hormone levels in urine that indicate the time the ovary is ready to release the egg. That meant they knew when to do the laparoscopy technique developed by Bob Edwards to collect eggs for fertilisation.

A press conference announcing the hospital's IVF programme was held outside on a patio and media from all the major television networks, radio stations and newspapers were there to cover it. Most of them were ignoring all the experts and eminent medical specialists, who could tell them all they needed to know about IVF and how it was changing the world. Instead they preferred to chat with me - just turned five years old I stood in a dress with mutton-chopped sleeves and told them about my dollies and what I did at school.

This became a pattern for my early school life. Most of the time I was just another South Bristol kid sat in class doing the usual things before going home to a fairly normal three-bedroom house and playing childhood games with my sister. Then every now and then I would be whisked off to do a media appearance or appear at some IVF event in some part of the UK and even abroad. Much of it I can't even remember. All the time the development of IVF meant there were continued moral dilemmas and each time Mum, Dad and me would be asked our opinion - usually Mum and Dad didn't have an opinion and as long as I said something cute people seemed to be happy.

Sometimes some money went into the Chandlewise account from these appearances but Mum and Dad were so grateful to Bob Edwards and Patrick Steptoe that if they asked them to appear on a programme or at Bourn Hall for an event they would invariably do it for them.

The number of different issues around IVF were perfectly illustrated when in October 1987, aged nine, I appeared on Wogan. At that time Wogan - hosted by the top BBC broadcaster Terry Wogan - was on after the early evening news. Our family travelled to London for the live appearance but Bristol hit the headlines that day for a different reason.

A man called Kevin Weaver, who had already beaten his mother and sister to death drove to a workwear clothing factory at the edge of Bristol with a shotgun with the intention of shooting his girlfriend. He killed two other people who tackled him before driving off and eventually being caught by the police after a chase.

All this was dominating the national news before the main BBC channel went over to the Wogan show, which that night was hosted by stand-in Sue Lawley and was an IVF special. Sue Lawley introduced the programme saying that in the past when a woman had a baby there was only one way it could have happened. But she pointed out that with the growth of fertility drugs, test-tube babies and surrogacy there was a moral argument raging once again.

First on were Neil and Susan Halton, who through fertility treatment had a multiple birth of seven babies. The babies had all died within 12 weeks of being born. They were quizzed on how they felt about the infertility drugs they had been given, why they hadn't decided to abort some of the babies to give the others a chance of life. All tough, and uncompromising stuff.

Next on was Kim Cotton. She had hit the headlines in 1985 as Britain's first commercial surrogate mother. She had been paid £6,500 to carry a child for an overseas couple who could not have children. The man's sperm had been used to impregnate her and she had been forced to leave the baby - dubbed "Baby Cotton" at the hospital after it was made a ward of court in the row over whether the whole process was legal. The courts had eventually agreed the baby could go to the couple who had paid Kim Cotton.

Then Sue Lawley talked about a "modern miracle" - me - and how there were now "4,000 miracles around the world" and introduced Patrick Steptoe. As a band played Brahms Lullabye he walked across the studio floor looking dapper in a blue suit and striped shirt, using a walking stick to steady himself. Mr. Steptoe was now in his 70s but still robustly defending his corner and putting all the controversy into context.

He said the term "test-tube baby" had been invented by the press as far back as 1969. He said he had wanted to help women because gynaecologists in the 1950s seemed to give the same treatment to every infertile woman and never seemed to look into the root cause of their problems.

Me, Mum, Dad and Natalie watched the interview on a television screen in an adjoining room. Well, to be honest, there were a load of other children there, all younger than me crawling and toddling around and I didn't catch much of the interview at all.

Suddenly a producer came and took me to the studio to stand at the side. Patrick Steptoe was answering all the questions. His breathing a little laboured under the hot lights. Sue Lawley was hitting him with all the moral questions. Why should so much money be spent on IVF when there are diseases and other things to cure she asked.

Said Steptoe: "Although infertility doesn't kill people it occasionally causes such unhappiness and desperation that people commit suicide. There aren't enough properly organised infertility centres to help people."

He was asked if he was somehow playing God. He replied: "Modern science and medicine is still a part of God's creation. There is no question of morality. We are not playing God. It is too serious to say we are playing God. It is just a continuation of the biological creation of God."

Sue Lawley asked if he feared a modern Hitler might take on IVF work and use it for the creation of some sort of master race.

He replied that he had been calling for guidelines since 1970 on the issue but no action had been taken by the Government. He was in his stride now. He talked about how it had been a team effort with Bob Edwards and others, how he called cloning "clowning" and then went through some of the crazier things that happened with the media around my birth saying he believed that there was a "mole" in the team who kept telling the press what was happening. Sue Lawley introduced a film of my birth and while it was playing I was led to the sofa and sat next to Mr. Steptoe, who gave me a reassuring look and patted me.

As soon as the film finished the camera came on to me and Sue Lawley said: "That's you Louise, have you seen that film before?" I nodded and she asked me if I knew who the man was sat next to me.

I said: "Yes - it's Mr. Steptoe. He made me." Patrick Steptoe told how we kept in touch with each other and then he held my hand as we crossed the studio floor to where Mum, Dad, Natalie and the other children and adults had been arranged around some sofas. The band played the Billy J Kramer song "Little Children" as me and Patrick Steptoe with his stick strolled across the screen on Prime Time television.

I sat next to Mum who had Natalie on her lap and Dad stood behind and Patrick sat next to me. Mum was asked how much Natalie had cost and she said she couldn't remember so they asked Dad, who also shook his head looking vague. Patrick Steptoe looked at his feet as Sue Lawley asked them if this was the last of their children and they said they weren't going to try again.

The spotlight passed to the others. A lady who had two IVF babies. They were biologically twins but because of the techniques used in freezing embryos they had been born at different times so were sisters - another miracle of science. Sue Lawley demonstrated just how much journalists understood the science by asking: "Have you got any other eggs in the fridge" - the poor woman looked confused and laughed.

By now the toddlers were charging around the television studio and Natalie was wriggling and one little boy kept shouting "Mum" over and over. There were 20 month old test-tube triplets with their mum Jane Kennedy, who explained about their birth in the increasing chaos.

Before the show ended Patrick Steptoe had just enough time to explain that he had now been responsible for 949 babies being born and that he hoped the 1,000th would be born close to Christmas.

The closing credits rolled and various people in headphones started disconnecting microphones; babies were being chased around the studio floor and in amongst all the chaos Mum and Patrick Steptoe smiled at each other. Sue Lawley had given Mr. Steptoe a good grilling and probed deeply but both Mum and Patrick Steptoe had been hiding secrets.

Firstly, Mum was once again under-going fertility treatment. When Natalie was just two years old she had contacted Mr. Steptoe once more and he had quietly ensured she had some tests and treatment at Bourn

Hall. It had not been a success. She was trying for one last time with some treatment being carried out in Bristol and some at Bourn Hall.

Mum never discussed these attempts with me and she always said that she was more than happy with her two children and her adopted daughter Sharon. I suspect though that because we were all girls she was trying for a boy. Certainly Dad would have liked to have had a boy to complete the family.

The other big secret was being kept by Mr. Steptoe. He had cancer. As I waved goodbye to him when we left that studio I had no idea that it would be the last time I would see the kindly, if slightly tetchy Grandad-like figure. I had just started to understand what being the world's first test-tube baby was all about. I certainly realised from Mum and Dad that Patrick Steptoe was a very special and wonderful person.

His genius had just started to be recognised. He had been awarded the CBE and earlier in 1987 he had been made a Fellow of the Royal Society. On March 21, 1988 Patrick Steptoe died.

Although he was such an important figure in my life my main memory of him was a little incident that happened when our family visited his home, where he had a swimming pool. As usual Natalie and I were having a bit of a battle and I saw my sister standing by the side of the pool and it seemed the ideal opportunity to get one over on her by pushing her in.

As I crept towards her with evil on my mind the voice of Patrick Steptoe boomed out: "Don't you dare". The power in his voice stopped me in my tracks. Patrick Steptoe was not the sort of man you messed with. Natalie stayed dry and I behaved myself.

Just at the bottom of the driveway of Bourn Hall is the little church of St Helena and St Mary. Built from field stones and ashlar from the 12th Century onwards, it has a twisted spire and a packed little graveyard. It was there that the family and friends of Patrick Steptoe gathered on March 30, 1988 to pay their last respects.

The management of Bourn Hall sent a car to pick us up for the funeral and as I walked down the little path towards the church I heard someone shout "Louise!" I looked around only to see a photographer hiding behind the trees and snapping away to get pictures of me.

All the national newspapers wanted pictures of the test-tube baby mourning the death of one of the men who had made her life possible. It was a sad occasion, especially for Bob Edwards and for Mum and Dad. Tim Appleton, Chaplain to Bourn Hall conducted the service and hymns "Praise My Soul the King of Heaven" and "The Day Thou Gavest Lord is ended" were sung.

The Bishop of Huntingdon, Gordon Roe conducted a burial in the churchyard where Patrick Steptoe was finally laid to rest. Part of the service made reference to the way some people had accused Mr. Steptoe of playing God. Elliot Phillip, an eminent gynaecologist and obstetrician, who had worked alongside Mr. Steptoe and Dr. Edwards, read a passage from Genesis.

It was the piece about how "God made man in his own image". Elliot Phillip, who was a friend of Sigmund Freud and who wrote a million-selling book called *The Technique of Sex* at a time when such a subject was difficult to get published, delivered the lesson from the front of the church. He had been at the Royal Society of Medicine meeting in 1966 when Steptoe had met Edwards and founded the British Fertility Society with them.

He ended his reading with the words: "The first commandment from God is also an invitation for man to join in his creation." Even at his funeral Patrick Steptoe was proving controversial!

Mum had been admitted for fertility treatment earlier that month. It had not been successful. She never tried again.

The death of Mr. Steptoe really marked the end of the pioneering days of IVF and some of the novelty-value that the world held me in. Bourn Hall Clinic, which he had founded with Edwards was in a strong position to continue and other clinics were opening up all over the world. The technique was being developed and new arguments over what drugs should be used, multiple births and other moral issues had replaced the controversies around my existence. In most countries the debate was now more over what was an acceptable way to carry out IVF and how far should the technique go rather than one about whether it should exist at all.

Because there were now more interesting new things for the press to write about surrounding IVF, coupled with our family's reluctance to co-operate, there was less media interest in our family. As a result Chandlewise Limited, set up when I was born, was doing little more than tick over.

Despite the telephone number figures that the press bandied about when I was born it had never been a big earner. Mum and Dad had owned 66% of the company shares with Paul Vincent holding the rest as company secretary and doing all the work necessary to keep the company going.

The first year of trading showed a total of £75,470 trading profit. The directors took out £14,000 and there was a whacking £20,600 tax bill as Corporation Tax was at 42%. Dad had got his car out of the enterprise on top of the monthly pay cheque.

In the early days it had been decided to buy some equipment that could be leased out to earn money. On the books it is down to "office equipment", I have no idea what kind of equipment was bought although Sharon believed at one time portable toilets were among the kit being hired out. The idea was that this would give a better return than simply getting interest on the money and would make the money work a little for Mum and Dad.

In 1980 income was £30,927, and over £10,000 of this was from leasing equipment. A total of £4,240 had come in from newspaper rights on my story and £7,615 on the book rights and a further £8,145 on television rights. That year Chandlewise returned a trading profit of £25,288, down by £50,000 on the previous year.

By 1981 income was down to £15,419, most of it - over £12,000 - coming from leasing equipment, just over £500 from newspapers, nothing for the book and £2,465 for television rights.

Natalie's birth in 1982 sparked renewed interest and income rose again to £23,397 with £4,800 from film rights, £4,750 from newspapers, £160 from television and £13,687 from leasing equipment. Mum and Dad drew just £7,000.

The books for 1983 show just £600 coming in from payments to do with media appearances out of a total income of £13,918, so again most of the money was from leasing equipment.

Similarly in 1984 there was just £750 that came in as a result of television rights on a turnover of £15,604 and Mum and Dad took out just £6,000. Some of the leasing equipment had got old and had to be disposed of or replaced.

Turnover halved in 1985 to £7,517 and all of it was down to leasing income. In 1986 it was £7,353, with just over £1,800 to do with television rights. By 1987 it was just £4,588 coming in from leasing equipment. It was all over. The accounts show just £50 paid in during 1988 and a decision was taken to close it down in May 1989. Chandlewise was dissolved three months later.

In truth in round figures the story of the world's first test-tube baby brought in around £110,000 over 10 years in media payments, some of which had to be paid out in legal fees, hotel fees and tax. It was a far cry from the £325,000 quoted by the Daily Express and others all over the world as the payment for the story about my birth. Mum and Dad had also spent so much of their time doing interviews, going on trips and losing pay at their normal work while the media acted as if they had just been handed a fortune for having a baby!

Of course to two people who had spent their early courtship sleeping rough in a railway carriage it had allowed them to have a nice home in a nice ordinary area and for that they were always grateful.

Just before I was born the Memorandum and Articles of Association of Chandlewise Limited were changed. I suspect Patrick Steptoe and Bob Edwards had something to do with it. Alongside the intention of managing media fees for Mum and Dad and myself it set out other aims.

These were:

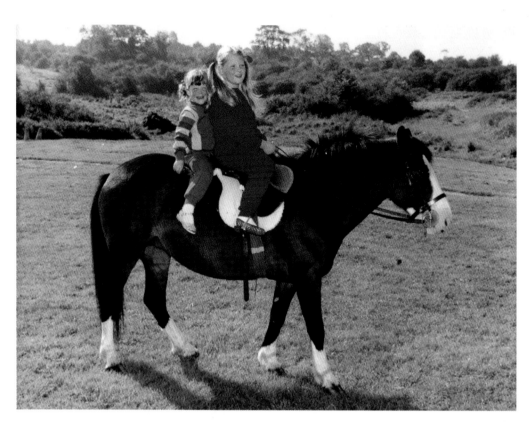

Me and my sister Natalie (top) taking a ride on a pony in the fields around our home in Whitchurch, Bristol and (below) playing in the garden

© Family collection

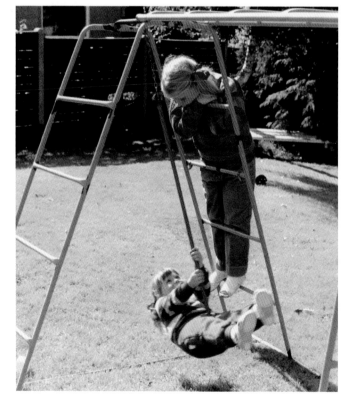

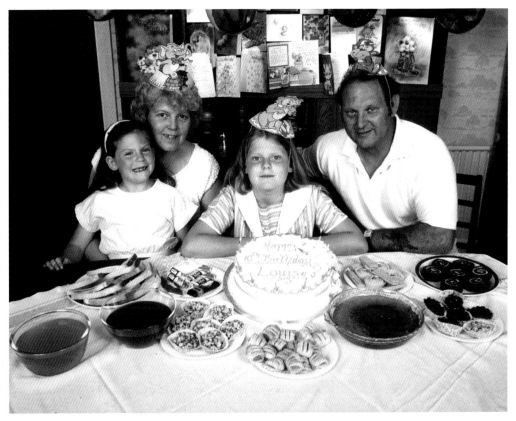

A family portrait on my 10th birthday...the media get interested whenever my birthday has a 5 or a 0 at the end! © Evening Post, Bristol

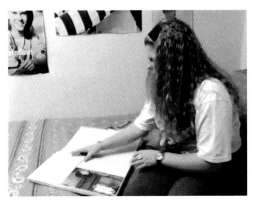 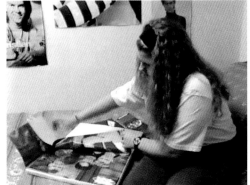

Whenever the media came to film me I insisted on showing them my Take That scrapbook. These are scenes from one of many documentaries. © TV stills

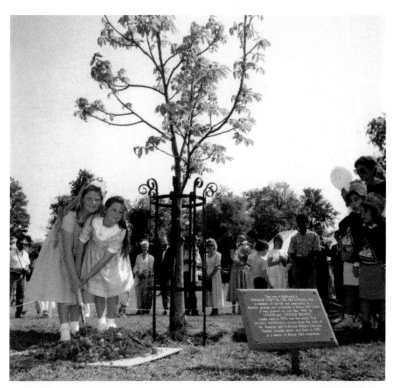

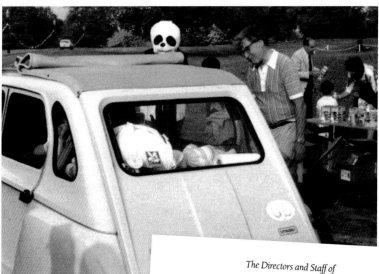

Natalie and I planting a tree at Bourn Hall, and Bob Edwards personally saying goodbye to every person leaving the first Bourn Hall Babies Party.

© Bourn Hall

The Directors and Staff of
BOURN HALL CLINIC
have great pleasure in inviting

MR & MRS BROWN

to attend the first ever
'BOURN HALL BABIES' GRAND PARTY
AND RE-UNION
Including a special tribute to Patrick Steptoe
from 2.00pm until 5.30pm, Sunday, 21st May 1989

R.S.V.P.

Dress: Informal

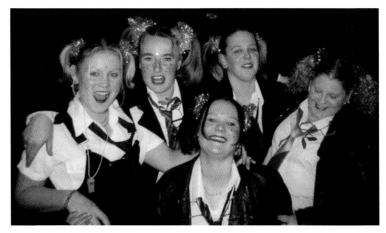

Staff from my first job as a nursery nurse, with me on the right. We all became great friends and still meet up regularly © Lisa Turner

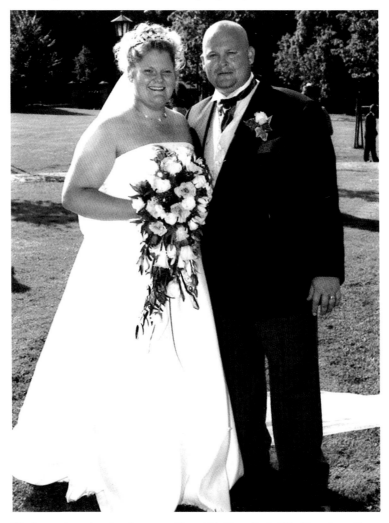

Wesley and me leaving the magnificent St Mary Redcliffe Church on the day I became Mrs Louise Mullinder © Family collection

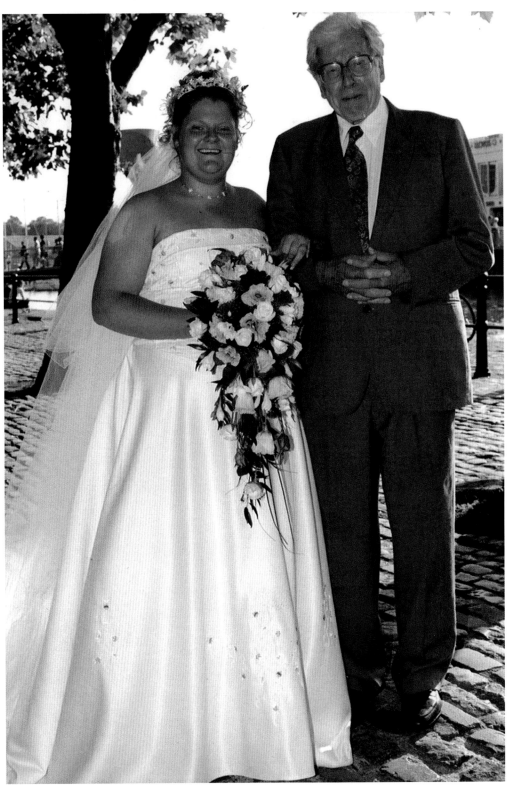

The photo that OK! Magazine didn't get. Me and a proud Bob Edwards outside my wedding reception on the harbourside in Bristol © Family collection

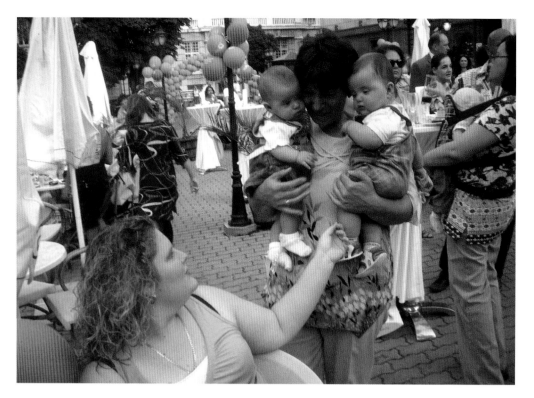

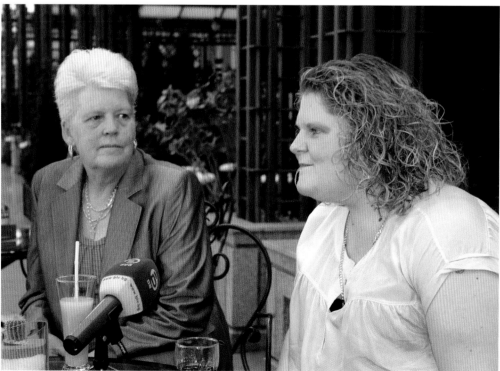

Our first visit to Bulgaria (top) meeting babies at a birthday party for me at a hotel in Sofia and (bottom) Me and Mum being quizzed by the national media in Bulgaria. © I Want A Baby Foundation

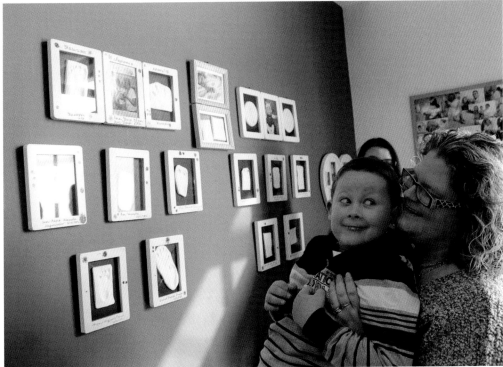

Our second visit to Bulgaria (top) a press conference as part of the Tree of Life conference and (below) Cameron was amazed to find his footprint on the wall of an IVF clinic in Bulgaria. © Martin Powell

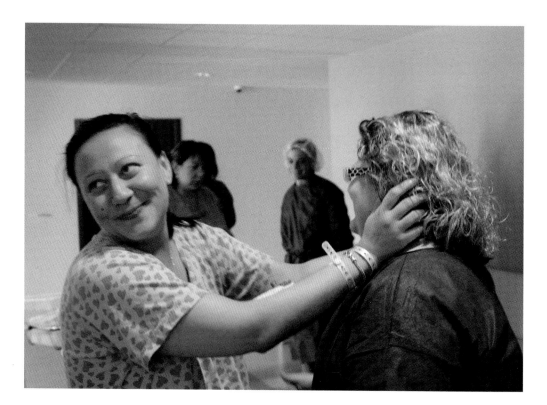

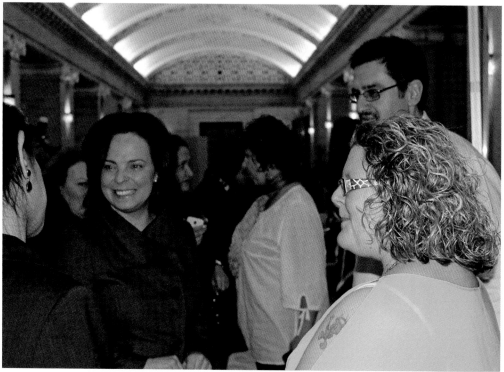

Top: A moving moment as a woman who had only moments earlier given birth to her IVF baby discovers that I was the first ever IVF baby. Below: Centre is Bulgarian Health Minister Tanya Andreeva at an informal moment during the conference. © I Want A Baby Foundation

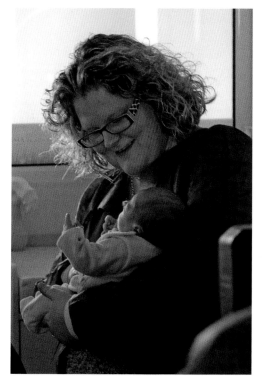
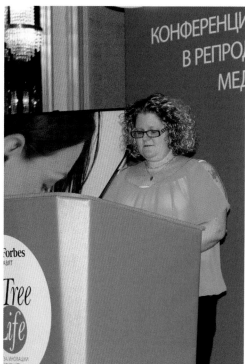
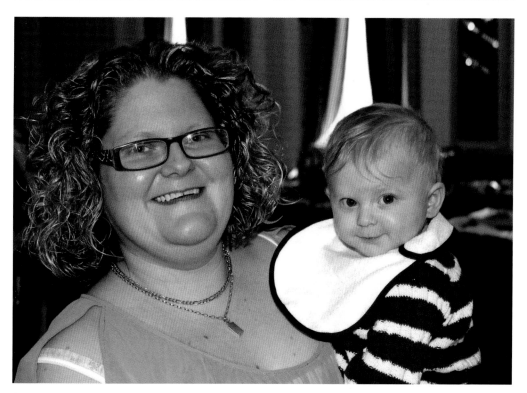

Top left: Meeting Bulgaria's latest IVF citizen just minutes after birth in the hospital. Top right: I give my first ever speech to a packed conference hall in Sofia. Bottom: Aiden enjoys the attention on his first experience of the IVF bandwagon. © I Want A Baby Foundation.

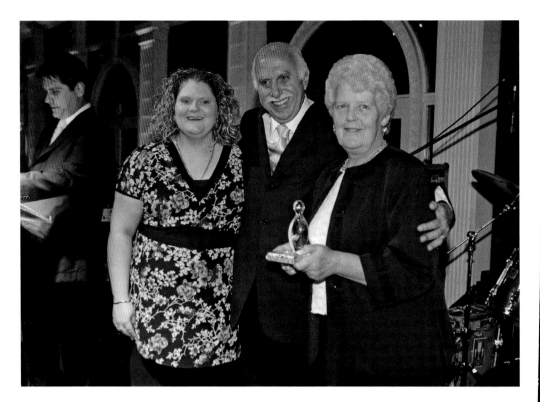

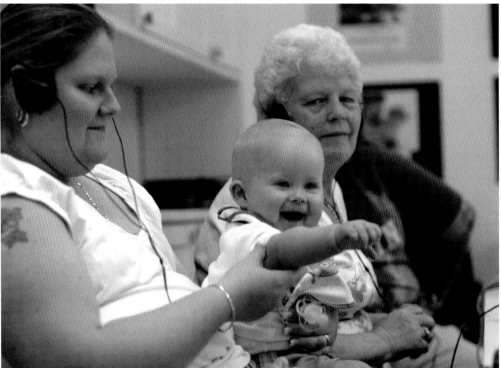

Top: In Brazil with Doctor Roger Abdelmassih, Mum and I received awards at a glittering ball.
Below: Facing the press in Brazil. Their questions were translated into headsets while Mum and I
kept Cameron entertained. © Clinic and Research Centre of Human Reproduction Roger Abdelmassih

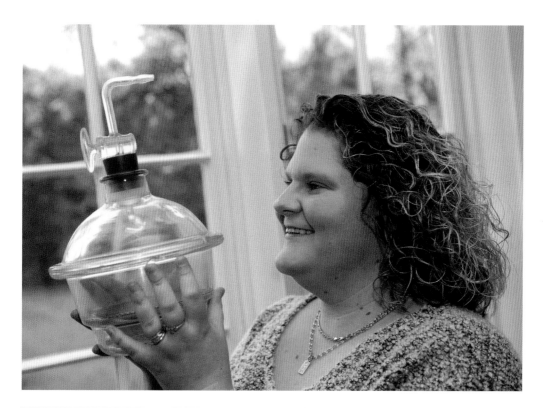

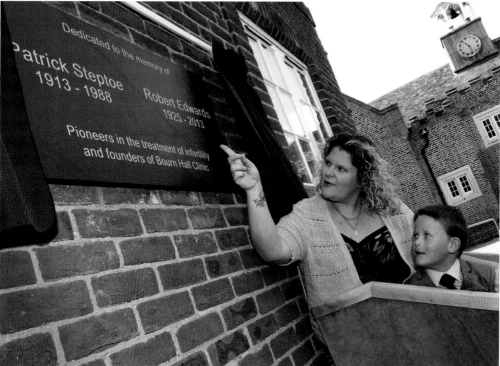

Top: This was the moment when I saw for the first time the jar in which my life began "In Vitro" and below: Unveiling a plaque to the pioneers at Bourn Hall with Cameron. © Si Barber

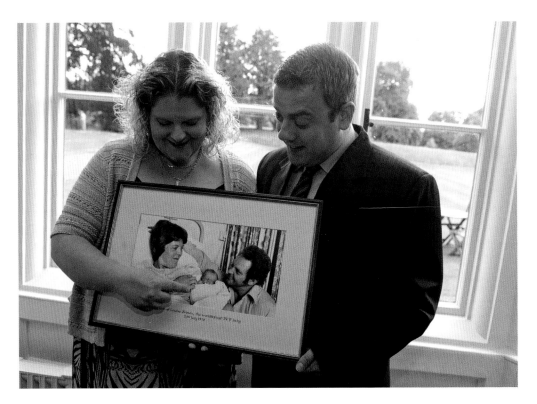

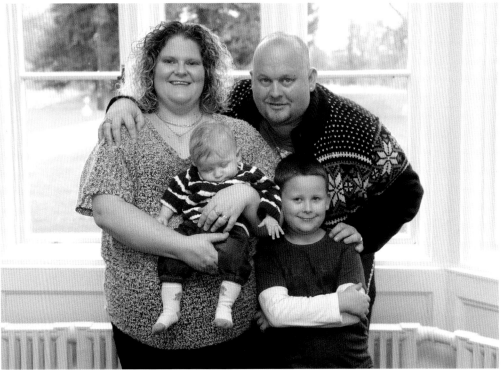

Top: Me and Alastair – the world's second "test-tube" baby with a photograph of Mum and Dad taken at my birth and (below) our family, my husband Wes and our children Cameron and Aiden.

© Si Barber

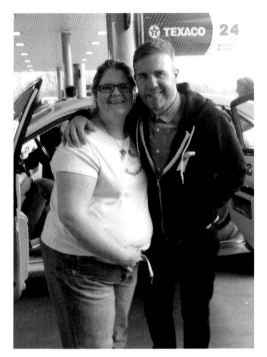
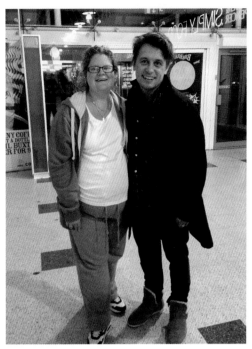

I have a habit of chasing members of Take That to service stations! Left: I caught up with Gary Barlow while he was raising money for charity. Right: Late at night after I had chased Mark Owen to Reading services while heavily pregnant and Sharon was in hospital. © Family collection

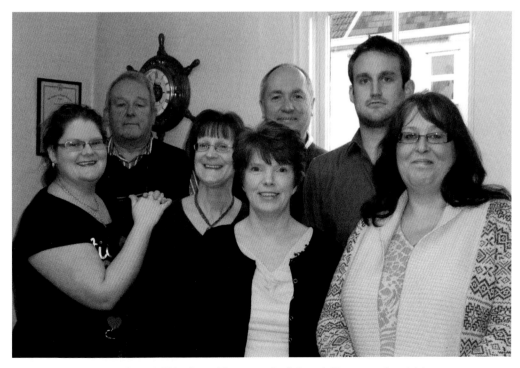

My work colleagues at Brunel Shipping with me on the left and Sharon on the right. © Family collection

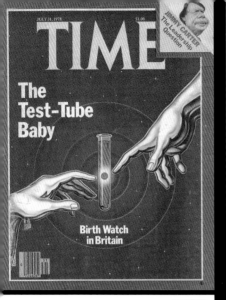

TIME

The Test-Tube Baby

Birth Watch in Britain

JIMMY CARTER
The Leadership Question

Evening News

Meet Louise, the world's first test-tube arrival

SUPERBABE

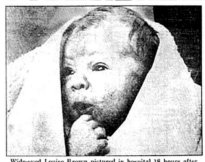

Wide-eyed Louise Brown pictured in hospital 18 hours after she was born. Today she's doing well. See Page Three

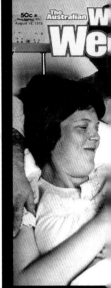

We

W

Daily Mail

£ MONEY MAIL TODAY

First test-tube baby is born and medical history made as a mother's dream comes true

IT'S A GIRL

Daily Mail Reporters

THE WORLD'S first test-tube baby was born last night — a 5lb. 12oz. girl.

She was nine days premature, and delivered by Caesarean section at 11.47 p.m.

For medicine it was a moment of history. For gynaecologist Patrick Steptoe it was a triumph of research. But for 30-year-old Lesley Brown, the tiny bundle that nestled beside her in Oldham General Hospital was suddenly less than a miracle.

And very today both mother and her husband baby were doing fine.

After nine years, Mrs Brown had given birth to the baby she longed for, thanks to the breakthrough by Mr Steptoe and Cambridge physiologist Dr Robert Edwards. Their achievement was to create life outside the womb — fertilising an egg with the husband's sperm in the laboratory and then returning it to the mother for a successful pregnancy.

Ritual

Mr Steptoe had decided to operate as soon as tests had shown the baby was supporting her own life. Lesley was overdue during the 9-38 minute operation.

With Mr Steptoe was his medical team and Dr Edwards. Lesley's husband, John, waited outside the delivery room, anxiously going through the experience. Lesley's chain-smoking ritual.

Mrs Brown, who had lost two babies in the maternity unit at Oldham for six weeks, was told only hours beforehand of the operation. The wait had become more tense, nerve-racking by the day. How had not been expected to give birth until August 8 and had to be in the hospital just she was the first test-tube mother.

The wait had become equally unbearable for her husband, who had been spending most of his time at her bedside. Yesterday he had been out shopping to buy Lesley a present for her 31st birthday next. Gerald Mendes.

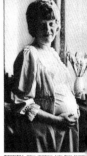

FIDUCIOSA Oldham (Inghilterra). Lesley Brown fotografata ieri

CHE RISCHI H

Il professor Arturo Giarola, eminente specialist
significato, i limiti e le incognite del metodo cli

DI CESARE CAPONE

---

woman

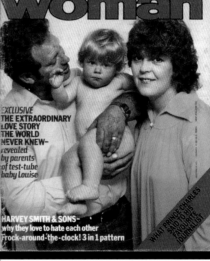
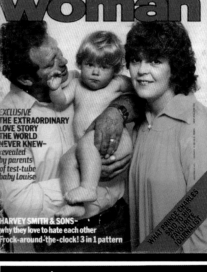

EXCLUSIVE
THE EXTRAORDINARY LOVE STORY THE WORLD NEVER KNEW—
revealed by parents of test-tube baby Louise

HARVEY SMITH & SONS—
why they love to hate each other
Frock-around-the-clock! 3 in 1 pattern

WHAT PRINCE CHARLES SAID TO HIS FAVOURITE JOURNALIST

---

stern

magazin

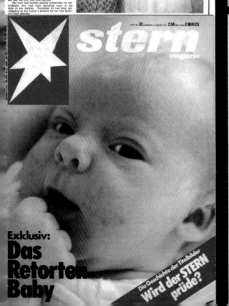

Exklusiv:
Das Retorten- Baby

Die Geschichte der STERN
Wird die STERN prüde?

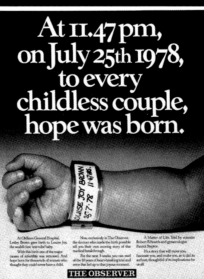

At 11.47pm, on July 25th 1978, to every childless couple, hope was born.

At Oldham General Hospital, the doctors who made the impossible possible tell you their own moving story of this medical breakthrough.

But the next 3 weeks, you can read of the 10 years of heart-breaking trial and error that led up to that joyous moment.

Now, exclusively in The Observer, the doctors who made the impossible possible tell you their own moving story of this medical breakthrough.

A Matter of Life. Told by scientist Robert Edwards and gynaecologist Patrick Steptoe.

It's a story that will move you, fascinate you, and make you, as it did its authors, thoughtful of its implications for us all.

THE OBSERVER

A Matter of Life. Starting on Sunday. Only In The Observer.

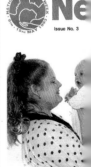

Happy birt

Louise inv celebrate a

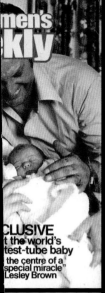

men's eekly

CLUSIVE
t the world's
test-tube baby
the centre of a
special miracle

Lesley Brown

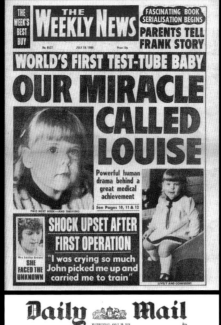

THE WEEK'S BEST BUY

THE WEEKLY NEWS

FASCINATING BOOK SERIALISATION BEGINS

PARENTS TELL FRANK STORY

No. 6521   JULY 19, 1980   Price 10p

WORLD'S FIRST TEST-TUBE BABY

OUR MIRACLE CALLED LOUISE

Powerful human drama behind a great medical achievement

See Pages 10, 11 & 12

TWO NEXT WEEK—AND THRIVING

SHOCK UPSET AFTER FIRST OPERATION

Mrs Lesley Brown
SHE FACED THE UNKNOWN

"I was crying so much John picked me up and carried me to train"

LOVELY AND CONFIDENT

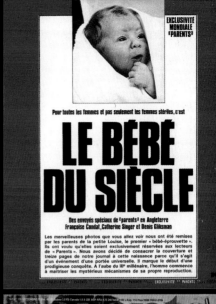

EXCLUSIVITÉ MONDIALE "PARENTS"

Pour toutes les femmes et pas seulement les femmes stériles, c'est

LE BÉBÉ DU SIÈCLE

Des envoyés spéciaux de "parents" en Angleterre
Françoise Condat, Catherine Singer et Denis Gliksman

Les merveilleuses photos que vous allez voir nous ont été remises par les parents de la petite Louise, le premier « bébé-éprouvette ». Ils ont voulu qu'elles soient exclusivement réservées aux lecteurs de « Parents ». Nous avons décidé de consacrer la couverture et treize pages de notre journal à cette naissance parce qu'il s'agit d'un événement d'une portée universelle. Il marque le début d'une prodigieuse conquête. À l'aube du IIIe millénaire, l'homme commence à maîtriser les mystérieux mécanismes de sa propre reproduction.

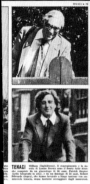

OGGI • 15

TENACI (Oldham (Inghilterra). Il marsupiale Patrick Steptoe

RSO LOUISE?

a della sterilità e collega di Steptoe, ci espone il
nascita della bambina concepita « in provetta »

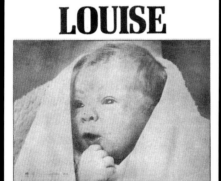

Daily Mail

WEDNESDAY, JULY 26, 1978   8p

And here she is...

THE LOVELY LOUISE

LOUISE BROWN, bright-eyed at 18 hours old: The test tube baby in hospital yesterday

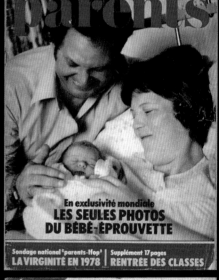

parents

En exclusivité mondiale
LES SEULES PHOTOS DU BÉBÉ-ÉPROUVETTE

Sondage national "parents-Ifop" | Supplément 17 pages
LA VIRGINITÉ EN 1978 | RENTRÉE DES CLASSES

"We won't be ignored any more" say Britain's angry would-be parents

1993

ALL SET FOR BIG AUNCH

campaign ready to go

o you!

to
ark

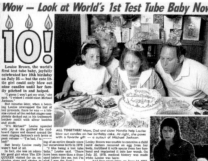

Wow — Look at World's 1st Test Tube Baby Now

10!

Louise Brown, the world's first test tube baby, joyfully celebrated her 10th birthday on July 25 — but the cute little girl could only blow out nine candles until her family pitched in and helped.

ALL TOGETHER! Mom, Dad and sister Natalie help Louise blow out candles on her birthday cake. At right, she poses with a favorite gift — a cutout of Michael Jackson.

FUNNY FACES: Louise and pal clown around with cake.

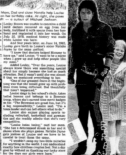

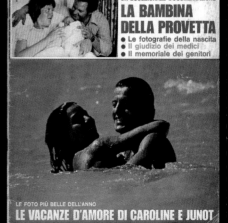

DUE GRANDI ESCLUSIVE

OGGI

ANNO XXXIV - N. 35 - 1978 - SETTIMANALE DI POLITICA ATTUALITÀ E CULTURA - SPED. ABB. POST. GR. II/70 - L. 500

UN'ECCEZIONALE DOCUMENTAZIONE

LA BAMBINA DELLA PROVETTA

● Le fotografie della nascita
● Il giudizio dei medici
● Il memoriale dei genitori

LE FOTO PIÙ BELLE DELL'ANNO

LE VACANZE D'AMORE DI CAROLINE E JUNOT

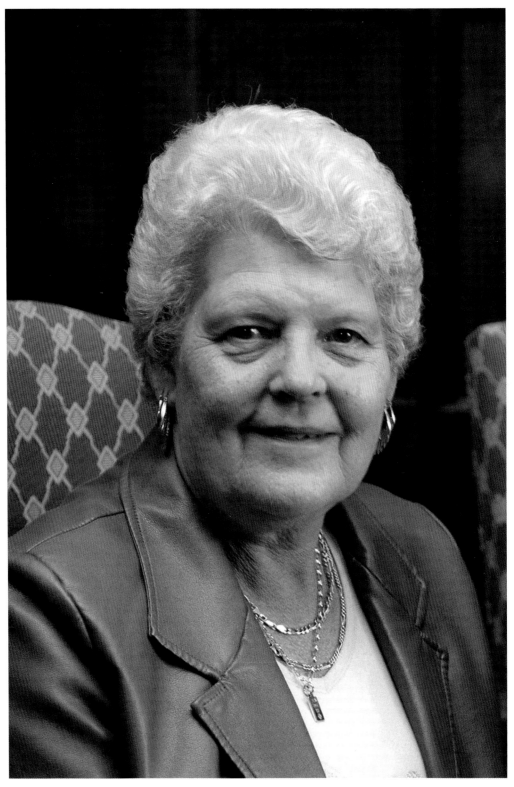

My Mum, Lesley Brown. An inspiration to thousands of women around the world. © Si Barber

"To further the advancement of research into the relief and treatment for persons who are suffering from disorders which give rise to infertility."

"To promote and advance medical knowledge of human reproduction, to develop new methods of contraception and sterilisation and to research into methods of preventing or alleviating genetic defects and to publish the results of such research.

"To establish a training centre for the purpose of teaching the advanced techniques which may be developed for the purposes aforesaid. To train personnel in such techniques.

"To establish a clinic for the treatment of such persons by such methods."

In reality Chandlewise never got involved in any of these worthy aims. They were all met by Bourn Hall Clinic and the Edwards-Steptoe Research Trust Fund. On Sunday May 21, 1989 I went to Bourn Hall for the first ever "Bourn Hall Baby Party", which was held as a tribute to Mr. Steptoe.

It was an overwhelming experience for me as a 10-year-old to suddenly realise what all the fuss was about. More than 600 of the 1,295 test-tube babies that had been created by the clinic were there with their families. As the oldest and the first everyone made a tremendous fuss of me and it was like being a fairytale Princess. Everyone knew who I was and all the mums wanted to have a picture of me with them and their baby.

Mum had picked out a pink summer dress and I had a headband holding back my hair. Most of the children were in party dresses and it was like a giant picnic in the grounds of the amazing house.

Bob Edwards spent a lot of time close to Mum and Dad, me and Natalie and was very emotional seeing so many families on the law celebrating the fact that they had children because of the techniques he had developed with Patrick Steptoe.

It was exciting for us children with party games, Punch and Judy shows, magicians, clowns and fire eaters and a marching band. There were pony rides and a bouncy castle and a giant party cake. The party started with yellow balloons, one representing every baby that had been created at Bourn Hall, being let off into the sky. They floated up into the blue sky, each with a ticket attached, and I was told later that the tickets were returned from Anglesey and Merseyside, some 250 miles away.

The weather was beautiful, as it often is at the end of May. Patrick Steptoe's wife Sheena was there and she made a lot of fuss of me and Natalie. It must have been a sad day for her to see such a celebration without her husband being there.

At one point me and Natalie were asked to plant a walnut tree in memory of Mr. Steptoe. It had already been put in place behind a plaque and they supplied us with one spade so there was the usual tug-of-war between us as we each wrestled to take hold of the spade and shovel some bits of mud on to the base of the tree while pictures were taken. Somehow, despite our sisterly pulling and shoving on the spade, each of us wanting to take control of it, they managed to snap some pictures where we look as if we are co-operating!

Not surprisingly the party had attracted the press, in a big way. tching us were an astonishing 160 journalists and 11 television film s from several different countries. Bob Edwards and his team and and Dad tried to make sure that they didn't interfere too much e and Natalie enjoying ourselves but all of them at one point r wanted to see me, talk to Mum and Dad and take pictures. ully there were plenty of other "human interest" stories rld of IVF there. An Icelandic couple called Gudjon had quads from 2,000 miles away for the party. Four little six y girls in frilly party outfits were always likely to draw he press and there were triplets and twins and others.

121

Bourn Hall had organised the event with a biotechnology company called Serono. It was the first ever big celebration of IVF and what it had brought to the world. At that time I believe the number of IVF babies had just topped 10,000, so amazingly a fifth of them were still the product of the work of Edwards and Steptoe and this particular clinic.

At one point a lady called Pat Pitcher gathered all 600 babies and children in one huge group on the lawn. Sat in the front, right in the middle were Bob Edwards, Mum and Dad and me and Natalie. The press wanted me stood at the front a few yards ahead of everyone else and of course Natalie wanted to be in the photo so we both stood there while hundreds of cameras snapped away. It seemed to take ages. Some pictures with Natalie, some without, some with Bob Edwards, some with Mum and Dad. The requests went on and on and I stood there with a fixed grin.

As the media snapped away and filmed I realised once again that this wasn't something that happened to anyone else. Just the day before I had been sat in class at school, no different to anyone else, now I was the centre of attention for the world's media, hundreds of people wanting to talk to me and be photographed with me and making a real fuss. It was absolutely crazy.

As the party broke up and started to leave there was a traffic jam forming on the drive. It was caused by Bob Edwards. Tears in his eyes he was standing shaking hands, and saying good luck to every single person as they left. Clearly moved at the sight of so many people whose lives had been changed by IVF techniques and obviously sad that his one-time partner Patrick Steptoe hadn't lived to see this day.

Along with Mr. Steptoe's widow Sheena he made a real fuss of me and Natalie as we were among the last to leave. It was the first ever party to celebrate test-tube babies and the photographs went around the world. There was no doubt that, although I might have been the first, this technique was now well established and there would be many many more to come.

I was finishing my Primary School years that summer and going to "big school". I really felt grown up. I had also become aware for the first time that my birth meant so much to so many people. They kept mentioning the word joy - my middle name - and for the first time I realised its significance. I wasn't a baby anymore but on that day I knew for the first time that I would be associated with babies forever.

Chapter 9

TAKE THAT AND PARTY

Hartcliffe School was a massive Secondary School within walking distance of our house in Whitchurch on the edge of the sprawling Hartcliffe Council estate. There were more than 1,000 kids in the school and those at the top end were more or less adults, many of them expecting to get jobs in the Imperial Tobacco Factory, which was the main place of work just a quarter of a mile away across a dual carriageway.

They seemed so big and old compared to us new kids starting. Imperial had built Europe's biggest cigarette factory in Hartcliffe. As a result just about everybody smoked as the workers there got free cigarettes, which they passed around their families. A big rust-coloured office block next to the factory was the company's international headquarters for those who were more suited to office work. For decades I think most people in South Bristol thought there was always going to be a job at Imperial or Wills Tobacco as it had been known before. After all smoking was always going to be popular, they thought.

But just as I started at the school the tobacco company announced the closure of the office block and a year later the factory closed with the production switched to Nottingham. It was a major blow for the area and the mood of the place changed as people found it harder to get work than ever.

To be honest I didn't really care much about what was going on in the area, or the world. My own little world mostly revolved around two new friends I made at the new school, Sarah Fisher and Becky Farthing. We just used to chat and hang out and listen to music and generally be pretty noisy around the place.

My first school report had my tutor saying: "Louise is just beginning to control her effusiveness which spills over in the wrong places all too often!! I am sure when she has learned to settle down a little more we shall see her helpful side emerging more."

My Maths teacher Mr Adlem wrote: "She does tend to chat rather too much" and my English teacher said: "Louise must learn to settle down much more quickly - she is very loud and bossy at present", while my Science teacher said: "Louise has settled in well, and apart from her chatter which occasionally gets out of hand, is working well in science."

I think from that you get the picture. I was noisy and loud and bigger than most of the girls and I suppose that is the answer to the question I so often get from journalists about whether I was bullied at school over being the first test-tube baby or whether it affected me in any way.

I can honestly say that it didn't and that was probably because I was noisier and brassier than most of the other kids around and bullies wouldn't have seen me as a potential victim. In fact a year later I was described as a "distraction" in maths and my science teacher wrote bitterly: "Louise is far more concerned with organising people than doing anything herself. As a result she does little work of her own."

There were some signs I was getting better though. My Physical Education teacher said: "Louise has calmed down during the year, but she still has a tendency to fuss with those around her rather than attend to the task in hand" and my tutor summed it up with "Louise is slowly learning to take her place with others in the class and let others have a say."

Hartcliffe School was a daunting place when you first went there but because I had come through all the years with the same group of friends that had been through Primary School with me they took little notice of my status as the world's first test-tube baby.

Just before my 13th birthday the history books will tell you that Hartcliffe erupted into three days of rioting. The area had just been overlooked for some Government funds that people thought would help the work situation that had been getting steadily worse since the tobacco factory had closed. The spark for the riots was the death of two local men, who had stolen a motorcycle and were killed when it collided with a police car. The heavy-handed actions of the police were blamed by many and they took to the streets for several nights, petrol-bombing shops and throwing stones at riot police while a helicopter buzzed in the sky constantly over the estate.

They were frightening times and I was kept in by Mum and Dad but many people thought that it was about time the south of the city got some attention - there was a feeling that all resources had gone to St Paul's after they had rioted in the 1980s. People felt it was the only way they could protest and try to get some balance back to an area that was really struggling. In truth most of the people going out on the streets at night were just going out to have a look at what was happening, usually attracted by the police helicopter. After a few days it rained and not so many people went out in the streets and the whole thing died down as quickly as it started. People also realised that far from grabbing the attention of the authorities they were just destroying the few facilities that we had.

As a thirteen-year-old girl I wasn't really interested in rioting or local politics. Me, Sarah and Becky were more interested in what was happening in the pop charts.

Sarah Fisher had gone to Bridge Farm Primary School in Whitchurch, so I hadn't known her before we met at Hartcliffe and Becky had come from St John's Lane in Bedminster a little further away but we found ourselves sitting next to each other in the tutor group at Hartcliffe School.

We used to play board games like Monopoly together in each other's houses and on a Sunday evening would often go to Sarah's house to listen in to the chart show together, taping off the songs that we liked.

Me and Sarah were really into Jason Donovan and we kept on and on at Sharon until she agreed to take us to Birmingham to see him in concert, as we weren't old enough to go on our own. By now Sharon had left the family home in Whitchurch and had a place of her own so sometimes I would visit my grown up sister.

Listening to the radio at Sarah's I remember we heard a new band called Take That and a song called *Promises*. We liked it and liked them even more when we saw Robbie Williams, Gary Barlow, Jason Orange, Howard Donald and Mark Owen dancing and performing on the television. At first they were just one of the bands we liked.

But then they brought out *It Only Takes A Minute* and along with most of the other girls my age I rushed to buy the CD and they got into the top 10. The bands on television seemed a long way away from our lives in Whitchurch but then we heard something amazing. Take That were coming to Bristol. But not just to Bristol they were coming to my little area of Bristol - Whitchurch!

The Whitchurch Sports Centre was an old aircraft hangar on the edge of the old airfield that had been converted to provide some sports facilities. Outside there was a running track and some five-a-side football courts and inside the space could be changed around for indoor football, tennis, badminton and other sports. Mum had taken a part-time job at Asda in Whitchurch and you had to walk past the sports centre to get to the supermarket.

We just couldn't believe that Take That were going to play within walking distance of our house. At that time they were doing lots of small venues all the way around the country and it certainly worked in building up the fan base.

With a little group of friends we got tickets and got right to the front on the barrier and I fell in love with little Mark Owen. Mark

Owen was six years older than me and was voted "The Most Fanciable Male In The World" in a Smash Hits poll - and honestly it wasn't just me voting!

But there was also something else exciting about him - he was born in Oldham - the same place as me. I didn't know anybody else that was born in Oldham so to my teenage brain it was a great thing that the two of us had in common.

Although the media kept knocking on the door, ringing up and sending letters Mum and Dad started turning down interviews that were simply about me and would only do things if it was to do with infertility or IVF, usually if Bob Edwards or one of his team asked us to take part. Around my birthday there would inevitably be reporters and photographers hanging around outside the house trying to get a picture of me.

Although my birth had shown that IVF techniques worked there was still a huge infertility problem in Britain and still a lot of people who didn't see it as a medical problem. They believed that if you couldn't have a baby, well, bad luck that was not something that precious medical funds should be spent on. A campaign had been going on for many years to make treatment for infertility available on the NHS. This led to the country's first ever National Fertility Week being held in May 1993 with events all over the country.

The week included the release of a survey that showed that treatment of infertility on the NHS was scant or non-existent in most areas. A petition was handed into the Secretary of State for Health as part of a lobby of parliament calling for more resources to be put into providing treatment for infertile couples. Events were being held up and down the country highlighting infertility as an issue.

What had once been a taboo subject was now being discussed openly and statistics showed that one in six couples in Britain might need some kind of help to conceive.

Of course the people organising the week of action wanted me involved and what they came up with was making me the guest of honour at a massive children's party for 8,000 people held at Thorpe Park near Chertsey, Surrey.

It was an exciting day for me and Natalie as the theme park had some great rides. Around 4,000 children, who had all been born through assisted conception were invited to the free event and they turned up with their mums, dads and brothers and sisters for the huge party with me at the centre of it all cutting a giant birthday cake and being the star attraction at a giant tea party on the lawn. Some of the children were babies just a few weeks old. Lots of the mums wanted their babies photographed with me and I just loved cuddling the little ones.

Ever since I had started at Hartcliffe School at the age of 11 I had thought that I might want to do some work with children. Now at 15 the pressure was on to decide on a career and on that day in Thorpe Park I became determined to become a nursery nurse. After all, I loved playing with the little ones and taking care of them.

The party organisers knew how to win me over. They presented me with a VHS video of "Take That And Party" that had been signed by the entire band - it immediately became my favourite possession.

Of course the press were there and they all wanted to interview me and ask me what my life was like and mostly I gabbled about Mark Owen and Take That. In fact in nearly every news story about me in those days Take That got a mention or I was posing in one of their T Shirts or pictured in my bedroom with their poster on the wall behind me. A reporter from People Magazine in the USA sent me a copy of a story and photos she had used with a little note saying: "Take That should be very pleased with all the publicity!"

The magazine, which featured Michael Jackson on the cover and a huge article on Telly Savalas gave me equal billing saying: "Louise Brown, the first test-tube baby, is now a 15-year-old Tom Cruise fan". The caption also says I'm a Tom Cruise fan but the picture is me and Natalie sat on a bed...I'm wearing a Take That T Shirt and on the bed is the book: "Take That Our Story"...I think the clues were there for the journalists.

London Tonight came to Bristol to interview me as part of a little series they did highlighting the problems of infertile couples. They showed me putting on the latest Take That single *Why Can't I Wake Up With You* and flicking through my scrapbook of Take That pictures cut from pop magazines. I told the reporter Clare Rewcastle that I intended to pass my GCSEs so that I could become a nursery nurse.

She also asked me how I felt about being famous and I simply said: "I ignore it. Sometimes it just gets embarrassing."

The exposure started the media bandwagon off again and the family were invited to visit the USA and Canada later that year as part of National Infertility Week there organised by their National Infertility Association - RESOLVE.

On September 30 we flew to Dulles Airport, Washington DC and were whisked off to Stouffers Concourse Hotel and suddenly from being an ordinary teenager in a school in Hartcliffe, Bristol I was once again touring the USA and making media appearances, this time for 10 days.

Mum and Dad had learned a lot from the early days insisting that a lot more free time was built in to the trip. But there was still a lot of travelling, media interviews and being in the spotlight at fertility events.

We had a sight-seeing tour of Washington DC and then went to the historic Union Station for an international reception put on by RESOLVE. Mum and Dad and me and Natalie were introduced to the convention made up of doctors, fertility specialists and people from the 58 groups all over the USA that made up RESOLVE. Bob Edwards and Howard Jones were among the people there.

Then it was on to New York where media duties included appearing on Good Morning America, being interviewed by the New York Times and on the telephone to the Los Angeles Times.

There was an event to celebrate the 10th anniversary of IVF in New York, held at the Columbia-Presbyterian Medical centre and a whole week of activities.

They picked us up in a stretch limousine and as it went around a corner Mum slid on the leather seats from one end of the car to the other - we all laughed so much. As a family we took a bit of time out to catch up with Christina Santiago and her family, who was now well-established as my American pen-friend.

We were supposed to meet Elizabeth Carr, the first IVF baby born in the USA but at the last moment we were told that she couldn't meet us.

Finally we went to Montreal in Canada where Bob Edwards and the Brown family were presented with the Barbara Eck Menning Award. Barbara Eck Menning had founded RESOLVE in 1974. She was a nurse who had set up a "hotline" to help infertile couples in her own home, after experiencing difficulties herself.

By the time we were in Montreal receiving an award named after her the kitchen-table helpline had grown to a nationwide organisation with over 25,000 members, showing how important the issue was in the USA.

Mum and Dad were told "You and your children have certainly contributed to a worldwide understanding of critical issues."

We made the long flight home with the award and instantly instead of being at receptions in the USA being applauded by hundreds of people I was back to being an anonymous schoolgirl at a Bristol Secondary School. My teenage years were punctuated by events like this.

By the time I was in my mid-teens I started going to "Nappy Night" at Ritzy's nightclub in Bristol. These were special nights for under 18s, where we could enjoy all the fun of being in a nightclub, except the alcohol.

Often celebrities from the television would be the draw for us. I remember the actor Les Hill, who played Blake Dean in the Australian soap Home and Away was there one night and me and my friends were queueing up to have our photos taken with him, after all he was a good-looking actor from the television about five years older than me.

There was also a band called Menergy that me and my friend Shelley got very excited about. They came to Ritzy's several times and we would be there drooling over them! We also used to go to the annual Balloon Fiesta at Ashton Court in Bristol every August where hundreds of brightly-coloured hot air balloons take to the skies. But, once again, we were more interested in the Thursday before when pop groups, including Menergy a band called Best Shot and others took to the stage. It was free too!

Mum and Dad agreed to more IVF events, but usually only if they met with the approval of Bob Edwards or involved a bit of travel to somewhere interesting. I assume they also picked up a little bit of money each time to compensate Dad for having to miss a few days at work or take days out of his annual leave.

In September 1995 we all flew to Paris from Bristol Airport on a Thursday for an international press symposium on new developments in the treatment of infertility, organised by Organon, a Dutch pharmaceutical company. We were met at the airport by the PR people and whisked to the Hilton Hotel in Paris and spent that evening and the next morning giving press interviews - all the usual questions for me and I suppose most 17-year-olds would be quite daunted by a massive press conference, but it all seemed very familiar to me as it had been happening all my life. The conference heard there were now 100,000 so-called "test-tube babies" in the world.

For me and Natalie the trip was about one thing - the organisers had agreed that once we had done our duties with the press the whole family would be treated to time at Euro-Disney and I'm pretty sure that's the only reason Mum and Dad agreed to do it!

Back home I'd started drinking, and smoking. I financed this and my social life with part-time Saturday jobs. I worked in Burger King for a while and Mum got me into Asda as a part-timer. Dad had moved on from driving lorries to driving buses, which meant I could get a free bus pass as a member of a busman's family, which also helped my social life.

My own close family was growing. Sharon, with her taxi-driver partner Kenny, had a daughter Rhiannon. We got a call one morning that she had gone into labour and Mum rushed to the hospital. I would have gone too but I had a shift at Burger King later that day and thought the birth would take longer than it in fact did. Before I set off to serve the burgers they were back to tell me about my new niece. Sadly Kenny died when Rhiannon was quite young and Sharon spent many years as a single parent. Rhiannon has always been a big part of my life.

I left school with enough qualifications to go to nursery nursing college in Lawrence Weston Bristol and fell in with another group of friends.

I spent a lot of time with Emma Trott. She lived on the other side of town so we would meet up in the centre of Bristol and travel together to the college.

We would ride on the buses at other times too and we would drink something called 20/20, which today I think I would hate.

Dad never realised it but we were often riding around trying to chat up the younger bus drivers and we would go into town telling our Mums we were each staying at the other's house so we could stay out all night or go back to people's flats and homes we met up with. It was all pretty typical teenage stuff.

I had a couple of teenage boyfriends. The first "real" boyfriend was a lad called Chris Buffery who I started going out with when I was 16. We met at the Cartwheel pub in Whitchurch and were friends for a long time.

The most serious one was Ian Perrett, who Emma and I met when we were riding around on the buses! He was a regular passenger, although he came from Plymouth originally. We got chatting and started a relationship that went on for about two-and-a-half years. I broke my heart crying when we split up but looking back it was a typical teenage romance.

The bus journeys often took us up Redcliffe Hill at the end of Bedminster on the way into the city centre and I would gaze at the massive spire of St Mary Redcliffe Church, the most spectacular church building in Bristol. With my teenage mates we would sometimes speculate on what it would be like to have a wedding in that church.

I left college with my Level 2 qualifications and got a job at Hampton Road Day Nursery in Bristol and my workmates there Laura Wood, Lisa Allen, Georgina Allen and Rebecca Chard became great friends and we would work hard and party hard. We still do when we get a chance to get together.

We would go to Liberty's a bar in Arno's Vale, Bristol and above it was a nightclub called Parkside where we would chat up boys, enjoy the music and do some terrible karaoke performances after a few drinks on a Friday or Saturday night.

Every birthday brought a round of media requests. It would be documentary-makers from Brazil, TV programmes from Japan and Germany, national newspapers wanting an exclusive interview, science correspondents writing features about the future. All would want to know what I was doing and what my views were on the latest developments in IVF.

Mum and Dad would pick and choose some to take part in if the people asked nicely or they felt they were helping Bob Edwards. But we didn't really have much to say. I had no idea what was going on in the IVF world.

My 16th and 18th birthdays were particularly hectic as the IVF community always seemed to choose the anniversary of my birth to launch initiatives and the press seemed fascinated with the "test-tube baby has now grown up" story. It was a little difficult at times and I had to be careful because it was obvious that the tabloid press especially would like any kind of nice juicy story about me getting drunk or seeing a boy or doing any of the normal things that teenagers get up to. I suppose the years of dodging them and watching my parents dodge them stood me in good stead.

Soon after my 18th birthday I had a tattoo on my shoulder of a shooting star. Mum didn't like the idea of women having tattoos and Dad didn't really approve, but he had so many that he couldn't really argue with me! My second tattoo was a heart and flowers and the words Mum and Dad on it - even though it was in tribute to them and all they had gone through Mum still wasn't keen - but they came from a different generation when tattoos were really something only men had.

Cheque-book journalism was still in full swing and my parents and me would accept money from the media when it suited us. We always saw it as payment for our time and inconvenience. Journalists don't realise just how disruptive their attention can be. They would say they just wanted a photograph and that would take half a day of your time as they messed around getting you to pose in all sorts of ways and then the result would be a tiny little picture in the paper.

They would say they wanted 10 minutes of your time for an interview but it was always an hour and then countless calls back to check something or to put words in your mouth because their news editor didn't think I had said anything interesting or exciting enough.

On my 20th birthday the South West News Agency in Bristol, who regularly sold stories to national newspapers wrote to me. Their features writer Fiona Locke offered me £5,000 for an exclusive picture and story if I ever had a baby. They said they would pay me £5,000 up front straight away and if I never had a baby then they would just write off the money. On top of that they would pay me a percentage of any money they made from selling the story.

It was quite ridiculous. I didn't even have a boyfriend at the time, let alone any idea that I might have a baby. It sounded like madness to be selling the rights to your future child and only a news organisation could think that was something a young woman might contemplate.

Also in the lead-up to my 20th birthday I had ABC television from the USA wanting me to take part in a one hour documentary about cloning, which also shows a lack of understanding. IVF really has little to do with cloning. My birth came about through the technique of bypassing the fallopian tubes and bore no relation to cloning.

So my 20th birthday came with lots of coverage all over the world. Little did I know until many years later about one consequence of this.

In Ireland a comedian called Brendan O'Carroll read an article about my birthday as he was heading into a radio studio. That day he invented a comic character. Needing a name for it, the article was fresh in his head - so he called the female character Mrs. Brown. Mrs. Brown's Boys later became a smash-hit television series. I had watched it many times before I learned that the family were actually named after me! What a strange life I have.

Chapter 10

MOVING ON AND MOVING OUT

As soon as she could Natalie left home and moved in with her boyfriend Lee Derrick. Lee worked on a farm in the countryside that surrounds South Bristol and was a couple of years older than me. It meant just me, Mum and Dad were at home again but I was spending most evenings out and chatting up blokes myself with my friends.

Just about everybody was on the contraceptive pill and I had been to the doctor and took up a form of contraception that involved having an injection every eight weeks or so. That seemed a lot easier to me than remembering to take a little pill every day.

It was called Depo and the doctor explained that one of the consequences of the injection could be that it would take more than a year to get pregnant after you stopped taking it. I wasn't really bothered about that. I was more afraid that I might accidentally get pregnant with some boy than I was worried about future motherhood.

It may seem strange but although all my life I had been surrounded by talk about babies, pregnancy and the struggles that Mum had been through I never really gave it much thought for myself. Of course from time to time I wondered whether I might have problems having children, whether Mum's problems could have been genetic. But I think until you are grown up and seriously thinking of starting a family it isn't something that really bothers most people.

I didn't have the slightest worry about taking contraceptive medication either. To be honest it was normal in the area where I lived when I reached that age for the girl to take responsibility and just about all my friends were on the pill or had some form of contraception lined up.

Certainly I knew that if I was going to have a baby I wanted to be in a relationship, probably even married, and make sure that we were in a position to provide for the little one. Nursery nursing had shown me some of the best and the worst of mothers.

It seemed Natalie wasn't quite so keen on contraception and she became pregnant while she was still 16. In fact her daughter Casey was born on May 13, 1999, just a few weeks before Natalie's 17th birthday.

It was only after the baby was born that the family discovered that Natalie was the first ever IVF person to have a child themselves - conceived naturally. So, my sister became a world first herself and we confirmed it with a trip to meet Bob Edwards, who by then was 73 but still keen to see another baby on the scene.

Bob Edwards pointed out the significance of the birth saying: "Casey is the icing on the cake of the IVF programme. In the early days people said babies conceived through IVF would be born with abnormalities or give birth to abnormal children. But we never believed that argument and now we are proved right. Casey is a delight and a charming little girl. Knowing that a young lady like Natalie has had a problem-free natural birth is wonderful.

"What we are seeing now is the second generation of IVF where children who were conceived by the test-tube process are moving on to parenthood. The fears that they may have been left infertile are completely laid to rest by Natalie's baby."

In fact all was not entirely well with Casey. She had a slight heart problem, which caused the family a lot of concern. Thankfully it was sorted out at an early age by the medical profession. It had nothing to do with the fact that Natalie was IVF.

The family's low profile at the time, which Mum and Dad had strived for by not co-operating with anyone much during our teenage years meant that Natalie's birth in Bristol and the problems with Casey's heart went unreported.

But of course I was about to be 21 and the media saw this as another milestone. Natalie and her partner Lee saw this as an opportunity to make a little money to help bring up Casey and through a friend sold the story to the Sunday People, who published it as a "World Exclusive" with a huge picture of Casey across the front page.

The media's appetite for "test-tube baby" stories had not died down in over 20 years as that newspaper proved by the fact that it chose Natalie giving birth two months earlier as the main story, giving it bigger coverage than another exclusive it had on Prince Andrew being secretly filmed having dinner with the glamorous wife of a millionaire and Eastenders actress and Carry On star Barbara Windsor photographed with a young lover.

The media still seemed to regard our family as a soap opera, just like the Royal Family was or the soap stars themselves were. The only difference was we had never asked to be famous and Mum and Dad were trying to keep out of the limelight. Casey was a great new addition to the family and Mum and Dad loved her dearly as the first grandchild to come out of the IVF programme, although they regarded Sharon's daughter Rhiannon as equally important as a grandchild.

Mum wasn't too impressed at Natalie getting pregnant and having a baby at such a young age but to be honest there were parallels with her own teenage years and I think Natalie was probably more like Mum was as a teenager than I ever was. Being in the spotlight so much probably made me a little bit more cautious with what I did. I was more interested in getting close to Mark Owen of Take That than anyone else and a letter through the post in advance of my birthday had made me hopeful.

It seemed that the borough of Oldham was celebrating its 150th anniversary and wanted me to go along as a guest for the celebrations. Surely, Mark Owen - Oldham's most famous son in my eyes - would get an invite as well?

We went up by train to Oldham and the local council put us up in the Hotel Smokies Park. The main event that they wanted us at was called "Oldham Innovation" held at the Queen Elizabeth Hall where people could learn about keyhole surgery, see a laser show and meet and talk to a robot. They could also see how the first test-tube baby was created with a talk by Bob Edwards and me making an appearance.

I also had an early birthday lunch with the Mayor of Oldham Councillor John Battye. It was a bit strange being guest of honour at a place that I didn't know very well but really Bob Edwards was using the event as a showcase for IVF and Mum and Dad were keen to support him in that.

Disappointingly there was no sign of Mark Owen and it seemed that the local council in Oldham thought I was more famous than he was! One significant thing for me was a visit to the Kershaw's clinic and Oldham General hospital where I was born.

My 20th and 21st birthdays had caused a frenzy of interest once again from around the world. The Japanese media got very excited about my 20th birthday as that made me an adult over there and they had seen little news about me since I had appeared there as a baby.

The 21st was of course the "key of the door" in the UK but Mum and Dad refused most of the media interviews on my behalf as they came in from the USA, Germany, Brazil and the Czech Republic. I told everyone that asked that I was going away for my birthday and it seemed the media believed it, especially after the Daily Mirror published a story saying I was spending my 21st birthday in Blackpool. In fact the landmark birthday passed quietly back in Bristol with a few drinks with my friend Becky, while national newspaper journalists searched the bars and fleshpots of the Northern resort of Blackpool hoping to find the test-tube baby behaving badly.

By now I was working at Asda in Whitchurch part-time on

Saturdays in order to earn the money I wanted to fund my trips into town and their national staff newspaper put me on the front page - but I didn't mind that as the store manager gave me a bottle of champagne for my troubles!

Requests kept coming in from all over the world - National Geographic wanted to do a piece on me; American documentary makers wanted us to fly to the USA. By now we were ignoring most things and often the media either contacted Bourn Hall, who said they would pass it on to us, or the local media in Bristol, who told people we were un-cooperative, as that was how they found us whenever they made tracks to our front door to ask for an opinion on something or other.

Far from being the recluse the media seemed to think I was I took a job that got me out and about a lot. I left the nursery and became a postal delivery worker. My round was the Hartcliffe council estate and I would be up early every morning to collect the letters that needed delivering and then walk around the estate pushing the letters through doors.

Apart from the odd yapping dog it was a job I absolutely loved. It was good exercise and quite fun and I got to know some of the people on my round. It is surprising what you get to find out when you are a post lady. Also important for me was that the job was over early in the day so it didn't interfere with my social life.

Emma and I used to drink in a pub called the Spotted Cow in North Street, Bedminster. Emma started going out with a guy called Mark we met there and we would all drink together along with a work colleague of Mark called John. John was gay and he and I hit it off brilliantly and the little group would go to John's flat or on to a club called the Aurora. The clubs all had doormen, or bouncers, as many people called them, to keep troublemakers out and restore order if anyone had too much to drink. We got to know the door staff at Aurora, a big girl called "Tabs" short for Tabitha, who sorted out any problems with the women drinkers and Simon, who could handle himself with any lads that caused trouble.

One day Simon announced it was his birthday and invited Emma and I to go out for a drink. We went to another club called Bennys. Of course a lot of Simon's friends were doormen, including those at Bennys.

Wesley Mullinder was on duty on the door at Bennys the night of Simon's birthday. I must admit I got very drunk that night so I don't remember much about the first meeting with the man who was to become my husband. Certainly, I have to admit, I used to chat up the doormen at the clubs and being friends with Tabs and Simon, always had something to talk to them about.

The next day, sobering up I went to Tabs and Simon's home in Throgmorton Road to have something to eat and Wes was there again. We got chatting and that led to us going out together a week or so later. We had our first proper date on March 25, 2002.

Wes working nights on the doors meant we could see each other in the day sometimes. In the evening I would usually go to the pub, where Tabitha was on the door. Then when she finished we would go together into town to meet up with Simon and Wes, who were often working on the same door as they worked for the same firm.

We saw more and more of each other and pretty soon I had joined Wesley's nocturnal world, where he started work at 10pm most nights of the week and worked until 4am when the last of the drunks had staggered home and the clubs closed.

Working the early postal round meant sometimes I then went straight to work and then crashed into bed in the afternoon so that I could be up to go and see Wes again the next evening.

Wes was a big guy. He had to be to ensure that trouble-makers and those who had too much to drink didn't get into the late night venues. Most of the time there was little trouble as all the clubs had their bands of regulars and people like Simon and Wes knew them well and knew who would behave themselves and who maybe needed to be reminded to calm down when they had drunk too much.

I can't ever remember telling Wes about the fact that I had been the world's first test-tube baby. Wes had a son Bobby through a previous relationship and he had been in trouble in his teens and we learned about each others lives as we got to know each other. He said he knew who I was that first day we met properly in Simon's home.

In fact it was no big deal in Bristol. Of course people had heard of me and knew my name but the fact that Mum and Dad had kept me out of the limelight in recent years meant that few people recognised me. Louise was one of the most popular names around at the time and Brown is a very common surname. Most of my friends knew about the famous start to my life but were far more interested in hanging out, drinking, getting jobs and all the normal things that people in their late teens and early twenties get excited about.

Soon I met Wes's family. Wes was living in the nearby coastal town of Clevedon in a flat with his brother Paul, so I met his brother first. His Mum and Dad were divorced and both had new partners. His Mum, Annette also lived in Clevedon with her husband Dave and they had a son Alistair. Wes also introduced me to his sister Mandy.

His Dad Cliff was married to his stepmother Pat, who had a son Michael. Cliff knew all about me as he worked for the local paper, the Bristol Evening Post. Cliff was a motorcycle messenger, riding his motorcycle around the region with vital things for the newspaper. That included unexposed film from photographers out on assignments.

In the days before digital technology and email he would stand by at the local football match and take the film from the photographers and rush it back to the photographic laboratory so that it could be developed and put into that day's paper. Or he would be in the press scrum outside court buildings on big trials waiting to take the reporters hastily scribbled words back to the newspaper to be set in pages for later in the day.

It meant he was well-known by all the journalists, photographers and cameramen of national and regional newspapers, radio reporters and television reporters. Often they would all be hanging out in the same place waiting for the story to happen. He had heard Louise Brown and her family were pretty un-cooperative with the media and whenever the name was mentioned it was usually followed by a moaning story from a reporter or photographer who had spent hours trying to speak to the family or get a picture organised only to be turned down.

He was fine with me and although he was part of the media circus that had chased me around for so many years it was never an issue between us.

In April 2003, just over a year after we first met, me and Wes got engaged. Of course my first thought was on how I could get St Mary Redcliffe Church - the one I had passed so many times on the bus - as the venue for my wedding.

I didn't do anything about it and months went by then one day I went to see Sharon and we chatted about whether the church would let me get married there. Sharon said the first thing they are going to ask is what date do you want to get married.

I hadn't really talked to Wes about dates - although he also thought St Mary Redcliffe Church would be brilliant if we could book it. Mum and Dad had always had the first two weeks of September off as holiday so that seemed like a good time to me.

Me and Sharon studied the calendar for 2004 and settled on Saturday September 4 as the ideal day for a wedding. I was too nervous to ring the church and in those days wasn't very good on the telephone. Sharon's job at Brunel Shipping involved a lot of telephone work, wheeling and dealing in sorting out freight arrangements for businesses all over the world. I persuaded her to ring on my behalf.

While I sat there she rang the church and after a few minutes put the receiver down and said to me: "You jammy bitch they have got that date free!" I jumped up and down in excitement but Sharon smiled and said: "There is just one problem. You and Wes have to join the congregation and go to church every Sunday for at least six months before they will finally say it is OK."

WORLD'S FIRST TEST-TUBE BABY

That didn't bother me too much but I wasn't sure quite how excited Wes would be at getting up early on a Sunday morning after a Saturday night on the doors outside the nightclubs. Saturday was always the busiest night of the week for him and he enjoyed his Sunday lie-in.

But I needn't have worried. The next week we joined the congregation and went to see the officials at the church and they booked our wedding date. Each week we would turn up and enjoy the service. On about the second week I spotted a girl called Gemma who also worked in Asda, Whitchurch where I was still working part-time to get a few extra pounds to pay for the wedding and our home together. It turned out she was getting married a few weeks after us and was also coming along for the same reason with her boyfriend.

We used to all sit together and listen to the service or giggle at Wes singing the hymns loudly. Sometimes Gemma would come along with her parents and our weekly trips to that beautiful church became quite an enjoyable part of our weekly routine as we started going to the evening service, which was easier with Wes's work shifts.

Of course to be able to get married in the church I had to become fully part of the church. I had never been Christened as Mum and Dad didn't go to church and felt it was hypocritical to have me baptised when they weren't particularly religious themselves.

So at the age of 25 I went into a little side chapel at St Mary Redcliffe Church with Mum and Dad and Wes for a short Christening ceremony conducted by the Reverend Tony Whatmough. Far from being a great significant moment in my life all I really remember about the occasion is that as the Holy Water was put on my head I looked up to see my Dad's stomach going up and down and wobbling uncontrollably as he desperately tried to stifle a laugh at my awkwardness. Mum was also grinning from ear to ear and Wes having to look at the ceiling to prevent himself laughing.

People with deep religious beliefs may find all this a little odd but really at that time there were few nice wedding venues like there are now and it was really a choice of a church or the rather dingy Register Office in Bristol. Many people did the same as we did and just got involved in a church for a year or so in order to have the service they wanted. Certainly the people at St Mary Redcliffe were very welcoming and we got to the stage where we looked forward to our church services.

In July 2003 I was 25 and of course to the press that was another landmark date - a quarter of a century of test-tube babies and once again in the lead-up to it letters from media people came flooding in asking for me and Mum to take part in interviews, television programmes and radio broadcasts.

BBC Woman's Hour wrote at the end of June wanting the whole family to take part in a broadcast. Another part of the BBC wrote the next day asking if Mum would be able to take part in a new series for Radio 4 called "The Reunion". The idea was that each programme would get a group of people together who had been involved in an important event and sit them down so they could chat about it.

They were planning to get Professor Edwards and others involved in my birth together for the programme and tentatively asked if I might speak to them. All the letters had the same tone about them, acknowledging that over the last decade or so the family had turned down just about every opportunity that had come their way.

In fact, considering we all worked for a living, there had always been a fairly constant stream of media appearances. Even if we didn't know about them my picture would pop on a programme or in a magazine article. Some of these latest requests offered money and Mum and Dad decided what we would co-operate with and what we shouldn't as we had the expense of the wedding coming up and wanted it to be as magical as possible.

Bourn Hall also decided to mark the 25 years with a baby party the day after my birthday and Mum and Dad thought that would be the best thing to do to support Bob Edwards. We appeared on BBC Breakfast TV on the day of my birthday and the media were out in force at Bourn Hall where some of the babies born through IVF had gathered to celebrate.

Once again I loved playing with the babies and meeting the other families and it brought home to me how much my birth was a symbol to childless couples of hope and potential joy - those two words that had followed me around all my life.

We did a press conference and posed for photographs and I told the media that really I just enjoyed an ordinary life and there wasn't much to report. I think my 25th birthday was the first time that Wes fully realised just how much interest there was in me. We had letters and requests from around the world and some publications were offering thousands of pounds. But often they wanted me to comment on things I knew nothing about - like the developments that were going on in IVF, the controversies over frozen sperm, whether women should be allowed to have babies from sperm belonging to partners who had died. They asked what I thought of the Catholic Church's attitude. They asked what I thought of certain pharmaceuticals or chemicals.

I was just a person who delivered the post in South Bristol and who worked in a supermarket at the weekend who was dating a hunky doorman and looking forward to getting married. I had no knowledge of all of this stuff and at that time in my life no real interest in finding out about it.

But the media wanted headlines like: "World's first test-tube baby slams Catholic Church" or "Stop the baby farms says first test-tube baby" or "It has gone too far says first test-tube baby."

I wasn't skilled at dealing with the media but from watching Mum and Dad I had become suspicious of them and had taken on Mum's attitude of being polite but saying very little. I'm sure some of the interviewers found it frustrating.

Of course they found it doubly frustrating if they had paid some money and still didn't get the story they imagined. I now realise that our attitude to being paid was a little different to the media. We just saw the payments as compensation for all the time and effort they expected us to put in for their programmes and articles. Often this would involve travelling across the country, dressing up, spending hours talking to people about the same thing over and over again or posing endlessly for pictures. Sometimes Me, Mum and Dad would have to lose out on our regular jobs to spend this time so we would be taking unpaid leave.

The media thought they were paying us for the story and content they had dreamed up. They expected us to co-operate with their questions, have an opinion on anything they asked and create the excitement for them to sell to their readers and viewers. Of course this was normal for them with regular celebrities, who had good reason to want to be in the spotlight. But we had nothing to sell to the public. The only financial advantage that might come from being in the public eye was another media organisation seeing it and offering us money to do the same again with them.

Wes realised that our wedding was going to be of huge interest to the media and we chatted about what we should do about it. Our first thoughts were to try to have the wedding quietly without the media being there. But they had already started asking questions about us and we knew some were trying to find out dates.

We talked to St Mary Redcliffe officials and they started to plan how they might keep the media out. They had a policy of having open doors on the church and said that part of the idea of a church wedding was that it was open for people to attend. Wes had his friends in the security industry and he talked to them about being on the doors on the look-out for media.

Sharon had a friend called Keith Biggs and Wes talked to him about our plans. Keith said that he would like to have a go at negotiating a deal with the media. We had learned from experience that it was impossible to do it yourself so we let Keith, who had no experience of such things, talk to some media on our behalf.

He rang round a few places and we went with him for a meeting in London with Express Newspapers OK! magazine and a deal was done for them to have exclusive rights to our wedding. The deal pretty much paid for the wedding but the main advantage to us was that they would provide us with a fantastic honeymoon - a Caribbean cruise.

In return they were given exclusive rights to photography at the wedding and the paperwork banned guests or anyone else taking pictures so I didn't bother booking a photographer for ourselves.

As the date neared I learned that their photographer was only going to do some limited pictures at the church so I spoke to them again and I booked our own photographer as there was a danger that our big day may not be fully captured.

Other media learned of the exclusive deal and were angry once again. We were being cast as money-grabbing individuals unwilling to share our big day with the world. In fact why would you let a lot of strangers from newspapers and magazines in to your private wedding just because they were curious about the way you had been born year's before?

The night before the wedding there was a rehearsal at the church and OK! magazine turned up in force with its own security guards who were checking that nobody was going to get coverage of the event.

The security team did a sweep of the church during the rehearsal and found a recording device strapped under a pew in the church. It had been put there by a rival magazine with the aim of getting the words of the ceremony the next day and putting it with some secretly snapped pictures. We were amazed that such a thing could happen.

The recording machine was near the back of the church so I don't think they would have got much from it but that find shocked and surprised the church officials and it was decided that once the ceremony was under-way the next day the doors would be locked to prevent anyone coming in. Some of the security people Wes worked with and some from OK! magazine would try to ensure that only our invited guests got a glimpse of me in my wedding dress.

The next day we had a wonderful wedding. The local news agency South West News, almost certainly prompted by one of the national newspapers, had a white van parked outside the church with a photographer in it and it was quickly spotted by the security people.

So when I arrived the people from OK! magazine used black umbrellas to shield me from that lens and ensure they had their exclusive.

My old security buddy Tabs spotted someone in the churchyard she didn't know and sure enough it was another journalist so she unceremoniously chucked him out by the scruff of his neck.

I walked down the aisle of the magnificent church I had always admired from the top of the bus with my bridesmaids Amber, Rhianna, Casey and Layla and my Dad looked so proud. There was a tear in Mum's eye and Wes and I exchanged our vows. The congregation sang *Lord of the Dance* and *Give Me Joy In My Heart* – two hymns we had enjoyed singing while being part of the church.

When Bob Edwards arrived the OK! magazine photographer stepped forward to take a picture of us together but Bob refused to be pictured saying the day wasn't about him. My photographer did take a picture of us together though, which I really treasure.

We had a car with a hood that came down and the original plan was for an open-top ride to a nearby hotel after the ceremony, but it was decided that with the photographers lurking around we would keep the hood up.

It is only a short distance to Jury's Hotel in the centre of Bristol so many of the guests decided to walk, including Cliff, Wes' Dad. As we set off for the church he saw the white van from South West News come along and walked in front of them on a Zebra crossing. He thumped the van window and told them in no uncertain terms to leave us alone and not to follow us. I think they were a bit shocked to see someone who they thought of as part of their own media circus turn on them and that was the last we saw of them that day.

I can't say the bit of press intrusion caused us any problems, really. The security and checking of names at the party afterwards all added to the excitement of the day. At one point I went to change my shoes and two security people escorted me to the hotel room just in case a photographer was lurking in the corridor waiting to photograph me in my dress.

My friend Kelly probably had more than a stressful time than me. Her friend had made the wedding cake and she had spent some time that morning balancing it on the pillars and was afraid it was all going to collapse on the floor. But she did a great job and we had a brilliant party at Jury's. My IVF family were also there.

Alastair, the second test-tube baby, now known as Alastair MacDonald, was there with his Mum. As a proud Scotsman he wore a kilt. Drinks flowed and the disco started and the DJ played party anthems.

By now I was just enjoying the day so when *Oops Upside Your Head* by the Gap Band came on I led our wedding guests in the "Boat Dance" which we all used to do to that record. That meant sitting down on the floor in a long line and by now I didn't care that I was wearing a white dress and scuffing it across the hotel dance floor. Alastair was equally excited and leapt down next to me and we all had a rather unexpected demonstration of just what a true Scotsman has under his kilt!

Following the wedding, despite a few worries about it being hurricane season, we flew to Miami for a few days then had a wonderful honeymoon on a Royal Caribbean Cruise liner and into the Gulf of Mexico.

For a while Wes and I had lived with Mum and Dad while we saved as best we could. But now married we moved into our own home in the Knowle area of Bristol. Not far from Mum and Dad and still in South Bristol.

Chapter 11

LIFE SERVES UP SOME SHOCKS

S oon after we were married I came off the contraceptive I was on. Although Mum and Dad's struggle to have children was well known all over the world I didn't ever really worry about whether I would have any difficulties having children and just assumed something would happen when the time was right.

Wes and I settled down to married life. Both our jobs were pretty low paid and neither of us very good with money. It was a bit of a struggle financially. Sharon had been working for many years at a freight forwarding company called Brunel Shipping and she knew of a vacancy that was better pay than I was on. It was a small business and she introduced me to the owner Phil Clayton and I started the job I still work at today. Sharon and I worked on different floors but it was good to see my big sister every day.

After two years I had still not fallen pregnant and on a routine visit to the doctors we chatted about it and I was told it was still likely to be the after-effects of the contraceptive. For the first time I wondered whether I might have to have some help to get pregnant if I was to have a family. To be honest I wouldn't have thought twice about going through IVF if I had to. As it happened I discovered I was pregnant a few months later. One of the first people I wrote to about being pregnant was Bob Edwards. I wanted him to hear about it first hand from me rather than when a press report appeared.

Dad wasn't well. Even at my wedding his breathing was laboured. He had been given an asthma inhaler and it had been put down to his smoking and lifestyle. Soon after we were married he had a heart attack and while in hospital suffered a minor stroke. He had recovered from that then suffered a second heart attack.

Just before I was due to go for my 20 week scan during my pregnancy the doctors diagnosed Dad with mesothelioma, a type of cancer that affects the mesothelial cells which make up the lining of the lungs. It is caused by small amounts of exposure to asbestos. Dad had worked with asbestos while driving for the railway company. He had been involved in projects working on railway tunnels, some of which had been lined with asbestos. His earlier breathing difficulties and heart attacks had all been part of the progress of his condition. Doctors said he had limited time to live.

I had no intention of finding out the sex of the baby but fearing Dad might not be around to see the baby born I asked him if he would like to know. He said he was confident he would survive to see his new grandchild and for me not to change my plans.

But as my pregnancy progressed Dad got worse and worse. The press found out I was pregnant and a story appeared. Wes suggested we should simply be vague about the dates to make sure they didn't start bothering us...so although the baby was due in December we told them January. As the due date neared it became apparent the baby was not going to move from its breach position and I would have to have a cesarean section. It was all booked for December 20 - just before Christmas 2006. We thought that having the baby so close to the Christmas holiday might keep the media away.

On November 29 Dad had another stroke and was rushed into hospital. He was in a bad way and for the first time I thought that maybe he would not live to see the baby born. We were visiting him every day and he was finding it difficult even to speak. He managed to tell Sharon about a ring that he wanted her to buy as a Christmas present for Mum. On December 6, from his bed in the Bristol Royal Infirmary he gave Mum that ring. It seemed a strange thing for him to do a few weeks before Christmas, but the next day he died, so I always believe that he knew his time had come.

None of us were with Dad when he passed away. Mum had been with me at the Maternity Hospital just a few miles away from where Dad was that morning and I had just dropped her home when Natalie called and said she had just heard from the hospital.

We all dashed to the hospital, including Dad's brother Keith, but he had passed away before we got there. He looked at peace and all his frown lines had gone. Dad's funeral was arranged for December 19 and Mum was convinced that all the trauma of Dad's death would send me in to labour, but we laid Dad to rest at South Bristol Cemetery and the next day I went into hospital and gave birth to a little boy. Wes and I had decided on the name Cameron a long time before but we decided to give the baby the second name John in tribute to my wonderful Dad.

As I held Cameron in my arms for the first time it was the end of an emotional roller-coaster. To have had Dad's funeral one day and to be celebrating a new arrival the next was pretty tough for everyone. In a way I think that Cameron's arrival helped Mum as she busied herself helping me cope with the new baby. She had been through all this before and was the perfect Granny to Cameron. I think he helped to fill the huge gap in her life left by the death of the man she had loved so much and been through so many things with.

The family rallied around and Sharon spent a lot of time with Mum over those next few weeks. Christmas was right on us and as everyone who has lost a loved one knows that can be a strange time of the year when it is the first Christmas without someone. Dad had always dressed as Santa when we were little and he had always been a major part of the Christmas celebrations. We missed him, but we also had the demands of a new baby, just days old, which changed everything for me and Wesley anyway.

The media had not found out about either Dad dying or Cameron being born so we were at least able to have that strange Christmas without them disturbing us. We knew that they would soon be making enquiries over the baby and during the holiday Wesley's Dad, Cliff, mentioned a former journalist he knew called Martin Powell, who was now a highly-respected public relations man in Bristol. His company represented lots of businesses and Cliff said he was trustworthy and would be able to help us deal with the media and maybe even get some money for the story of Cameron's birth. We were still struggling and now I was on maternity leave my earning power was limited. Work for Wes had been tougher in the last few years and we also had all the things that we needed to buy for Cameron. Our cars were on their last legs and it had been a year of disruption and problems.

Me and Wes went to see Martin Powell at his offices, which were a converted barn in Long Ashton and straight away we hit it off. He was from South Bristol and could remember when I was born and knew all about my story. We took Mum along to a second meeting and she liked him too. He had a small staff of friendly people and we agreed that he should handle all media enquiries from now on for us and try to get some money for us when he could.

As a result Cameron's birth was announced in an exclusive story with the Mail on Sunday, who also did a deal with News At Ten so that it was a major item on that programme on the Saturday night before the paper was published. Martin fixed up all the interviews and did all the arrangements for us and even hosted the photography and interviews at his own home to keep the press away from our house. When the photographer from the Mail on Sunday didn't like the clothes we were wearing he provided a jumper for Wes and his wife Mary, who was a similar size to me, supplied me with a blouse - so we appeared cuddling Cam in the national media for the first time in clothes borrowed from our PR man!

Having help to deal with the media was really important as it took the pressure off us and Mum, who also talked publicly about Dad's death at the same time. The story in the Mail on Sunday sparked a flurry of interest from the rest of the media around the world and Martin and his team at his company, Empica, dealt with it. Since then if any media want anything from me they have to talk to him first! It has saved so much hassle.

As we settled in to coping with having a baby for the first time - with a lot of support and help from Mum requests continued to come in from all over the world to Martin.

In Brazil Dr Roger Abdelmassih was the best-known IVF specialist. He had treated a string of high-profile clients and had hit the headlines in South America when he had helped the legendary footballer Pele at the age of 55 father twins with his second wife. Abdelmassih was a pioneer of IVF treatment in Brazil and had met Bob Edwards on many occasions and they had exchanged information.

His successes had included helping the former President of Brazil Fernando Collor become a parent and helping top television stars and celebrities have babies.

He had a fantastically successful IVF clinic in Sao Paolo and had gained celebrity status in Brazil, appearing with all the stars of that country and top politicians. The clinic included a stem cell research laboratory that was also carrying out leading work in pushing the IVF techniques forward.

Dr Abdelmassih was a star in Brazil and he did a lot of marketing and publicity to keep himself in the limelight. In August 2007 his PR adviser, Angela Arantes got a call from him. He felt business needed a boost and he set her the task of coming up with an exciting marketing campaign or story that would push his clinic back into the headlines and which would promote IVF.

Like all good publicity people she looked to see if there were any anniversaries near and realised that November 2007 would be exactly 30 years from my conception in the petri dish. Of course that date of

November 11 had never really been publicised much, people tended to focus on the date of my birth as the main anniversary.

But Angela was actually right - the real pioneering and breakthrough moment for science had been in that moment when Jean Purdy had seen the cells splitting on that November day. Angela set about trying to trace me and found Martin Powell. Her idea was for me to attend an event in Brazil on that anniversary.

After some negotiation Martin did a deal that meant that not only would all our expenses and loss of earnings be covered but that after the IVF event we would all have a nice holiday in the Brazilian resort area of Bahia. Unlike the days when I was little we wanted to ensure that flying halfway round the world included some leisure time and a chance to at least enjoy the sunshine of South America. It was fixed up for me, Wesley and Cameron then 11 months old and Mum to all fly out to Brazil, make some public appearances then go to the resort for a holiday. The year following Dad's death had been tough for us all, especially Mum, and we all appreciated the chance to have a sunshine holiday in a place we would never be able to afford ourselves.

Dr Abdelmassih knew the publicity value of my first ever visit to Brazil and he organised a banquet at which I would be guest of honour. Invited were celebrities, doctors and the media. It was also arranged that we would all appear on a television programme called Fantastico, which was one of the most-watched TV magazine shows. During the broadcast I would meet with the girl who was the first IVF baby ever to be born in Brazil.

Unknown to us two days before we were due to land in Brazil and while we were packing our bags and getting ready to go to Heathrow Angela Arantes received an email which was to change Dr. Abdelmassih's life. The long email claimed that Dr Abdelmassih had sexually abused a woman who had gone to him for treatment and had twins. The anonymous writer said that he or she would go to the press in the next few days and reveal the doctor as a sexual predator on women.

As you can imagine with a high profile visit from me just hours away, prime time television slots booked and a celebrity banquet all planned with some of the best-known names in Brazil this was a pretty shocking email for a public relations adviser to receive. Those close to the doctor had a meeting and pressed ahead with the plans for our visit worrying that it could all blow up into a scandal while we were there.

We arrived in Brazil blissfully unaware that this was going on behind the scenes and at no point did we get any inkling that there were any worries. We met Dr Abdelmassih, who was a charming man to me and Mum. He insisted on paying for us to buy some new clothes for the formal banquet and paid for everything during our stay in Sao Paolo including some photographs that I had done of Cameron.

He had a glamorous young wife, who we met, and his grown up daughter, a biologist called Soraya and son Vincent, from a previous marriage, who also seemed to be playing important roles at the "Clinic and Research Centre of Human Reproduction Roger Abdelmassih", which he had founded.

There was no doubt that Dr Abdelmassih was in charge and was held in high esteem by those around him. The first test-tube baby in Brazil was a beautiful 24-year-old woman called Anna Caldeira. She was a lovely girl and our meeting was stage managed for the television cameras as planned with Dr Abdelmassih introducing us.

There was a press conference with me and Mum listening on headsets to an interpreter, who translated the media questions from Portuguese to English while Dr Abdelmassih stood proudly on the sidelines.

Our visit to Sao Paulo ended with the banquet attended by 450 people - I'm told some were among the richest and most famous people in Brazil. Once again I was centre stage and both me and Mum received awards from Dr Abdelmassih on stage. Again, another odd moment as an ordinary girl from Bristol and her Mum end up on the other side of the world being applauded by hundreds of complete strangers, some of which experts in their field, to celebrate the 30th anniversary of being conceived!

After the banquet Dr Abdelmassih hugged me and Mum and thanked us profusely for our visit before arranging for us to catch internal flights to a lovely holiday-resort, where we were able to relax and enjoy the sunshine, all expenses paid. It was good for Mum to have a far away holiday and Cameron enjoyed some of the animals we encountered. At breakfast time monkeys came down and stole croissants from him as he sat in his high chair and we had an amazing family day out at a turtle sanctuary.

Nothing happened during our visit over the allegations about Dr Abdelmassih but a month later another email was received at his clinic and soon an online blog was set up about Dr Abdellmassih with people making claims about misconduct involving him.

Then a social media campaign about him started on the Brazilian social networking site Orkut and soon the scandal broke. Those close to Dr Abdelmassih knew that he enjoyed his celebrity status. He bought all his clothes in Paris, he ate at the finest restaurants, where often people would ask for his autograph. He was certainly a womaniser and he had a number of affairs.

Within months of our visit the story broke in the Brazilian media after he sacked a female receptionist at his clinic and she claimed sexual harassment. The media campaign led to prosecutors in Brazil finally looking into some of the rumours and stories that were circulating on the internet and in the same way that we have seen a number of celebrity sex scandals in Britain Dr Abdelmassih was arrested and questioned.

He always denied all the charges but in November 2010 he was convicted of a string of offences involving the sexual abuse of 39 of his patients, including three of rape. He was sentenced to 278 years in prison - the longest ever prison sentence handed out in Brazilian legal history at that time.

The court case was sensational with stories of the doctor sexually interfering with women while they were unconscious during IVF treatment of him using his position of power to sexually interfere with women and many different stories about his sexual behaviour.

It was a story in Brazil as big as the Jimmy Savile scandal in the UK. But it didn't end there. The doctor launched an appeal and was released from prison pending that hearing. In 2011 he disappeared along with his glamorous wife. It is believed that he slipped across the border into Paraguay. In August 2014 he was found living in a luxury house in Paraguay and taken back to Brazil. An appeal against his conviction is still in progress.

I have no idea of the rights and wrongs of what happened in Brazil. While there I got to know people close to Dr Abdelmassih and they maintain to this day that he was not a rapist and sexual predator. They do say that he was indiscrete and his own young wife was someone he had an affair with when she came in to have IVF treatment. On the internet it is easy to find the other side of the story and the people who say their lives were ruined by him. I guess nobody will ever know what really went on.

When I visited Brazil that country had just celebrated the fact that over 6,000 babies had been born through IVF as a result of the clinic set up by the doctor. It is shocking that a person who had seemingly helped so many people had fallen from being a rich celebrity to a convicted criminal.

Chapter 12

"I WANT A BABY" IN BULGARIA

S o having celebrated the 30th anniversary of my conception in South America I was expecting to spend my 30th birthday quietly at home with my cheeky one-year-old son and maybe a few family and friends.

But those plans all changed when Martin Powell was contacted by the "I Want A Baby Foundation" in Bulgaria. When I was born Bulgaria was part of the Eastern Bloc and somewhere my parents would never have dreamed of ever visiting in their lifetime and was certainly not a place that they would go with their new baby.

Little did they know that the news of the birth of a baby by this strange new method had reached into the Balkans and had been remembered by many people for so many years. The "I Want A Baby Foundation" had been formed in March 2007 by a campaigning lady called Radina Velcheva as a non-profit making, non-Government organisation with the aim of helping infertile couples.

It was estimated at that time that there were 130,000 infertile couples in Bulgaria and Radina had got together a powerful lobby of people, including doctors, biologists, psychologists, artists, public figures, journalists and couples who had successfully been treated for infertility issues.

Most couples who couldn't conceive in Bulgaria didn't seek medical help and, although there were experts in assisted reproductive treatments many couples simply felt ashamed of being infertile. Bulgarian men especially didn't like to admit they were having problems and were unlikely to talk about it with anyone. Not being able to have children was not a subject that people would discuss openly in public.

But Bulgaria itself also had a problem. According to the United Nations it ranked fifth in the most ageing population in the world. People aged over 60 made up almost a quarter of the population, whereas for most of Europe it is around 11 per cent.

In their first year of operation the foundation had made great progress in raising awareness among Bulgarian people and starting to change perceptions so that people were no longer afraid to admit they were infertile and instead started to seek the help they needed.

But they needed a catalyst to help make an even bigger impact and they decided that I could be the one to help them. In discussions with Martin Powell it was agreed that I would visit Sofia with Mum and attend an IVF seminar at which some of the most important people in the industry and the Government would discuss the problems and stigma of infertility. At first they wanted me to give a speech but I really didn't feel qualified to talk about the industry. In the end it was agreed that I would say a few words of greeting and Martin would give a little talk on how my birth had changed attitudes around the world.

We flew from Heathrow Airport not really knowing what to expect from a country we knew so little about. Me, Mum, Wes and Martin spent most of the flight passing Cameron from lap to lap and trying to keep him happy and then the plane circled the Balkan mountains and out of the window we got our first glimpse of Sofia as we slowly descended. But just at the point when we expected to hear the wheels bump onto the runway the plane banked steeply upwards and flew on over the terminal building.

Everyone on the plane looked at each other. The calm voice of the pilot then announced "The more observant among you may have noticed that we didn't actually land at Sofia. I'll be back in a few moments to explain it to you but just at the moment I'm a little busy."

It was rather typical British understatement. I'm always a little nervous on landing and take-off in planes and so is Mum and we both looked at each other starting to worry as the plane circled round. Martin leaned over and said: "It's OK for you. At least you will be the headlines in the paper if we all die in a crash. I'm just going to be anonymous." Mum winced but we all laughed nervously.

The plane circled round and the pilot explained that the wheels hadn't locked down properly and he was going to try them again. We heard the clunk as they were brought back up and then a noise as they went back down and we started to descend again. This time we hit the runway as normal and applause broke out throughout the length of the plane. Out of the windows you could see fire engines on standby. It was a shaky start to our Bulgarian adventure.

We got our bags and walked out into the arrivals hall at Sofia Airport only for Martin to be laughing again. There was a small group of attractive women with flowers and bright balloons attached to them. One had a sign saying "Martin Powell" and another a sign saying: "I want A Baby". Our PR man said it wasn't a welcome he was used to getting when he travelled.

We were whisked to the Grand Hotel Sofia where we had a suite for me, Wes and Cam. The wonderful team from the "I Want A Baby Foundation" were great hosts. The first night we all went to a local restaurant where we sat outside. Sofia was basking in 100 degree summer heat and it seemed so hot to us that it was nice to be outside in the evening. We met Dessislava Raitcheva, who we immediately started calling Dessy, who did so much of the organising and arrangements with the media. The wonderful Radina was central to everything and made us feel so welcome.

At that first meal Martin chatted to Radina's husband Bodgidar, who he nicknamed "Bodge" and after a few glasses of the local Rakia we all felt we had made some great friends in Bulgaria and we started to get a little bit of an idea of the importance that was attached to our visit to Sofia.

The next day was just as hot and after breakfast Me and Mum got ready for our first public appearance while Wes looked after Cameron and Martin went to the function room in the hotel where he discovered the conference had a slogan that read: "30 Years Louise Brown Thank you for the hope!"

Dessy and her team were busy placing dozens of press packs on seats ready for the press conference, each bearing the slogan. The pack even included postcards with a picture of me, Mum and Cameron on which had been produced in case anyone wanted our autographs.

The foundation was brilliant at getting publicity. For two years it had produced a television programme dedicated to the subject of fertility problems, giving the latest information about treatment to the public. Some of the top fertility specialists had appeared on it.

The foundation had also joined forces with a bank to provide financial help for couples so that they could borrow money to have a baby if they needed it for the treatment. It had also launched a programme providing psychological support to couples, especially women, who were affected by the fact that they couldn't have children. In some ways the work of the foundation was far in advance of what was happening in the UK - we were surprised.

Martin said it was important we all arrived together at the press conference. The hotel lift was small so we squeezed in around Wes's bulk and the pushchair with Cameron in it. The photographers and television people somehow realised that we were about to appear and rushed into the lobby... so the first view the people of Bulgaria got of us as the lift doors slid open was Wes's backside in his tracksuit and next to him Martin trying to climb over a buggy in his suit. We all started giggling and went into the packed press conference.

There were so many television cameras and they were all so interested in Cameron that we had to take him to the front to sit on the main table, alongside Bulgarian IVF specialist, Dr Georgi Stamenov and

Radina. We followed the proceedings through an interpreter and we answered questions from the media for an hour or so.

Then there were a whole series of other interviews to be done with television in a lovely little garden at the back of the hotel. Martin and Wes were able to keep Cameron occupied, although he was enjoying the fuss being made of him by Dessy, Radina and many other Bulgarian women. Mum and I answered the questions as best we could about our lives with Mum able to encourage Bulgarian women to take the step and have treatment if they needed it.

That night we were taken to a wonderful Bulgarian-themed barbecue centre in the hills where we met Dr Georgi Stamenov and his wife who had set up a clinic in Sofia. They had been at the press conference earlier but at the meal we had more time to socialise and get to know them without the media spotlight on us. There was folk singing and dancing and Martin and Bodgidar and Wes got stuck into the Rakia before the meal and as darkness fell coals that the meal had been cooked on were spread upon the ground and some spookily-dressed dancers appeared and started dancing on the hot coals. It all seemed very odd and incredible to be in the foothills of the Balkan mountains watching people walking and dancing on hot coals.

Next day we were up early and rushed to Bulgarian National television where we appeared on their breakfast programme. Me and Mum spent a little time in make-up and the idea was that we would sit by the presenters while Wes and Radina Velcheva would sit on the sidelines and contribute if called upon. It also meant Wes could look after Cameron if he squirmed too much! As it was still over 100 degrees and he didn't expect to be on TV Wes was wearing a short-sleeved T-shirt showing the tattoos on his arms.

Mum told her story through an interpreter saying: "After the operation to unblock my fallopian tubes didn't work we thought surely if men are going to the moon they can do something for us." She admitted that she felt desperate at the time and would do anything to have a baby. I got the usual questions about what it was like growing up in the spotlight then much to his surprise Wes found himself being quizzed by the presenter.

We didn't realise at the time quite how significant it was for a big bruiser of a man like Wes to be on Bulgarian TV and to say casually that if there had been any problems in conceiving Cameron he would have been quite happy to go through IVF treatment. The camera zoomed in on the tattoos on his arms and it was the perfect cue for Radina to talk about how the Government should help Bulgarian men and women and how people should speak more openly about their problems.

Mum explained that IVF babies were now just a normal part of society in the UK and said she hoped that our visit would help to solve the problems in the country. We were taken in cars back to the hotel where Martin, now understanding what our hosts were trying to get from our visit, delivered a speech to a packed conference that included health professionals and members of the Government.

Then we were off to a nearby park for another television interview. They wanted to film Cameron playing on the swings and despite the fact that the play equipment was graffiti strewn and in poor condition we did the interview, although I don't think any British TV stations would have used that backdrop for a story about babies.

That evening our hosts had planned a fancy dinner for us at one of the best restaurants in Bulgaria. Dr Stamenov and his team and representatives from the international pharmaceutical company Merck, who make many of the drugs used in IVF treatment, were attending.

The restaurant had fish swimming in a tank that people chose to eat. Wes doesn't eat fish and Mum didn't fancy anything and I had Cameron with me so it all got a bit awkward. Every time our guests looked away Mum slipped a bit more food on to Martin's plate and he manfully ate for all of us. It highlighted the problem we have of people thinking we are celebrities when really we would have been happy to go to a much more modest eating place. We felt very out of place and the meal didn't really work either for us or for our hosts.

The next day we went in a minibus to the IVF clinic run by Dr

Stamenov and we chatted to some of the women there and Mum really enjoyed playing with the babies and chatting with the women. While we were there one woman said that it was a superstition among many women in Bulgaria that if they touched me it might help them to get pregnant. It explained at last why so many of the women we met wanted to hug me or just wouldn't let go of my hand when we met.

We had some free time in the afternoon and Martin spotted Dessy, Radina and her team making all kinds of preparations out of the back of the hotel. A stage was erected and huge arches of balloons were put up. It was a surprise birthday party for me.

We walked out to enormous applause from a big crowd of people that had gathered, many of them with their babies. The stage had my name on it in huge letters and the words "Thank you for the hope." A massive birthday cake was produced and live butterflies were released by women, making wishes for the future and hoping to have babies.

It was incredibly moving with women bringing their babies to be photographed with Mum and me, many with tears in their eyes thanking Mum for being a pioneer and thanking us for enabling them to have babies of their own. Then a whole parade of Bulgarian pop stars started performing in our honour and we were invited on stage to have flowers presented to us and more speeches.

The people started dancing around as the cake was handed out in a sort of Bulgarian conga. We had little idea what was going on but it was a joyous celebration and party. Then everyone lined up for a massive group photograph with me and Dr Stamenov and Cameron at the centre of it all. It was an amazing last night to our stay in Bulgaria.

During the proceedings Martin came over to me and said: "Louise you realise this just doesn't happen to anyone else. Nobody else in the world has a massive birthday party thrown in their honour in a country they have never been before with top pop stars and hundreds of people they don't know attending."

But what was even more remarkable is the effect the visit had on so many people in that country. Mum and I were a real catalyst for change. During the visit the Bulgarian Ministry of Health agreed to look at the idea of establishing a state fund to reimburse couples for up to three IVF treatments in either public or private clinics. The Fund for Assisted Reproduction was duly set up in April 2009. Of course it was the work of the Foundation over many years that got the result but the visit by me and Mum had brought it to the top of the national agenda.

We went back to Bulgaria five years later to learn that 11,600 reimbursed IVF procedures had been carried out by then and more than 3,000 babies born. On top of that more than 22 Bulgarian cities had set up funds to help the treatment of infertile couples - the money adding up to around £750,000.

The "I Want A Baby Foundation" had gone from strength to strength organising amazing cultural events that helped to promote IVF and assisted reproduction.

On our second visit both me and Martin spoke at the Tree of Life Conference. The Bulgarian Health Minister Tanya Andreeva started proceedings speaking to an audience of almost 500 people about the "demographic problem" that Bulgaria faces and how IVF was playing its part in ensuring the country had a future. She explained that measures were needed to try to halt the decline of the country's population, which was continuing as people left to seek their fortune elsewhere and as an ageing population was not producing babies.

Then it was my turn. It was the first time I had ever stood at a conference of this type and delivered a speech. Martin had written it for me a few weeks before and I had practised in front of Wes but seeing so many friendly faces in the audience it wasn't as nerve-wracking as I had feared. Then Martin gave a talk on how the world had changed since my birth and pointing out some of the moral and religious challenges that my birth had brought to the world. He talked about same sex couples having children, using IVF, in a country where same sex partnerships had not been formalised in any way; outlined how IVF was allowing women to have children later in life and many other aspects that started the debate for the day-long conference.

Television and radio interviews followed and the next day we visited the amazing new clinic that had been built by Dr Stamenov since our last visit to Sofia.

The Nadezhda Clinic has been purpose-built as an IVF Hospital and was quite stunning. I was amazed to find in the corner of the huge atrium which is used as a central waiting area pictures from our first visit and a plaster cast made then of Cameron's feet and hands on display alongside other significant babies from the clinic's history.

Always good at publicity the team there had timed my trip to the minute and at 1pm the hospital was exactly one year old and I had reached the canteen where staff and couples going through treatment had gathered. A cake with fireworks in it was brought in and there was a question and answer session held.

I learned that people were travelling from Germany, Ireland and other parts of Europe to have treatments at the clinic. We saw the treatment rooms and all the latest equipment that is used today in the huge range of IVF treatments and techniques.

Up in the nursery some babies were sleeping. They had been born that day and we went in to see them, Cameron was really keen to peer into the cots and see the tiny little new-borns.

At that moment a woman came down the corridor wearing a hospital gown and pushing a trolley with a tiny baby in it. It was obvious from the way she was walking carefully and the exhausted but smiling look on her face that she had just given birth.

She came across our little party, complete with television cameraman following us around, and walked past us to put her baby into the nursery. One of the nurses explained to her what our strange little group was doing there and who I was. She rushed across to me and threw her arms around my neck and started kissing me and saying over and over "Thank you, thank you. You were the first, without you I would not have had a baby."

It was an emotional moment and finally she released her hug and held my face between her hands and said: "This is the happiest day of my life. To have my own baby is the greatest gift. Thank you."

We all had tears in our eyes and it brought home to me what my birth means to so many people around the world. I realised as we toured the hospital that maybe I can use the fact of my birth to help others and to raise awareness of the sadness of infertility and also the great joy - there's that word again, my middle name - that having children can bring.

My feelings on that trip to Bulgaria had maybe also been affected by the things that had happened to me in the five years since my previous visit. They had certainly been traumatic and eventful times.

Chapter 13

THE PIONEERS

It had been a dramatic five years between our first trip to Bulgaria and the second. Events in my own private life and in the IVF world had really brought home to me what my birth meant to so many people. I suppose Mum and Dad had always been so matter-of-fact about it and had protected me so well that I had never really thought of the significance to the world of being the world's first test-tube baby.

Mum received some money as a result of Dad's death through asbestosis and announced that she would like to use it to take the whole family on a special holiday to Florida. Ten of us flew into the USA on my 32nd birthday in 2010 with Natalie and her children, Sharon and Rhianna and me, Cameron and Wes. Things started to go wrong as soon as we got to the airport terminal.

Wes is a rough, tough bouncer and in his youth he hadn't exactly been an angel. He had a court conviction against his name and the details of the offence hadn't been properly filled in on the visa forms that they need to get into the USA so he was taken off by the security people for questioning when we arrived at the US immigration desk while the rest of us sat around waiting and hoping that he would be allowed to enter the country.

Mum found it all pretty stressful but after a couple of hours Wes was cleared through immigration and we travelled to the hotel. Mum was breathing badly and at first we put it down to the Florida July heat and the stress at the airport. She got worse and before we had been in the USA for 24 hours Mum was admitted to hospital with breathing difficulties and she was given checks.

The American hospital was brilliant and it was all covered by insurance but it meant the first week of our holiday was traumatic popping in to see Mum, who after all was paying for this holiday and was spending it in a hospital bed. She had imagined that this would be the last great gift from Dad, paid for from money received because of his industrial illness, but we were spending so much of the time visiting her and worrying about the medical checks.

Natalie's youngest child Daniel was a baby and needed to be looked after and the stress of the situation showed when Sharon and Natalie had a big row. It certainly wasn't the sunny happy family trip that Mum had imagined when we booked it!

The hospital checks revealed a shadow on Mum's lung and we all feared that she might have cancer. She was discharged from hospital after seven days and able to join in the second week of the holiday but it was still all pretty subdued worrying about what might be the result when we got back to the UK for more tests.

Back at home she had further checks and was diagnosed with emphysema. She started to use puffers to help her breathe but otherwise seemed to be able to get on with her life as normal. Sharon, who in her usual way had been the leader of us sisters as we had fussed over Mum for the first week of our holiday, went to the doctor herself a few months later with some health worries but the diagnosis was not so good - she had breast cancer.

I remember when Sharon told me the news with the words: "Well, we spent all that time on holiday worrying that Mum had cancer and now it turns out I'm the one who has developed it!"

As usual Mum rallied round and supported Sharon who went through a series of treatments battling against the cancer. Here we were all grown up but still Mum was our main support - looking after Cameron for me while I was at work, helping Natalie and her children out and supporting Sharon through her medical treatment by going to the hospital with her and just being there.

Better news came in a telephone call one day from Bourn Hall. Robert Edwards was about to receive the Nobel Prize in Physiology or Medicine for 2010.

I knew enough about the Nobel Prize to realise that it was a pretty amazing thing to get. I was also surprised that only now - 32 years after my birth - was Robert Edwards being recognised for the genius work that he did.

The press release from The Nobel Assembly of Karolinska Institutet told how more than 10% of couples worldwide are infertile. It talked about my birth as starting a new era in medicine and the millions of people worldwide that had been helped by the techniques.

The last line of the press release said: "Louise Brown and several other IVF children have given birth to children themselves; this is probably the best evidence for the safety and success of IVF therapy. Today Robert Edwards' vision is a reality and brings joy to infertile people around the world."

I have no idea what prompted the Nobel Prize people to at last recognise Bob for the work he had done but if Cameron's birth played a part in that then I am pleased. Certainly it was very very sad that they left it so late to honour Bob in this way. He and Patrick Steptoe faced so many obstacles and only now was the world realising what a benefit their work had been for so many people. People literally owe their lives to them. They wouldn't be here if they hadn't pioneered the technique.

Although I was pleased at the award I was also aware that Bob was not in the best of health and not able to go to collect it. If only he had been honoured 10 years earlier then he might have got the moment of glory and pleasure that he richly deserved. Now as a frail old man he was unable to do any interviews or speak about the world acclaim he was at last getting.

I'm sure it was a proud day for his wife Ruth and his daughters to go to the spectacular Nobel Prize ceremony and receive the honour on his behalf.

It was an odd moment for me too. The press asked for comment and I said some nice words about Bob and expressed my feelings about how over-due the award was. Once again I was able to think how strange it was to be an ordinary person living in a modest house with my family working every day at a shipping agents in Bristol and suddenly my very existence had resulted in a Nobel Prize being awarded.

I was just an ordinary working mum. Every day while I was at work in the offices at Brunel Shipping my Mum was, like many other grandmothers, doing a fantastic job of looking after Cameron during the day at our old home in Whitchurch. Each night after work I would drive from the office in Stokes Croft in the centre of Bristol to Mum's house in Whitchurch to pick him up.

Once he started school, either me or Wes would take him in the morning and then either Wes or Mum would pick him up in the evening. On the days Mum picked him up she usually looked after Cameron at her house until I finished work. It meant that Cameron was used to going to his grandmother's house a couple of times a week and playing there. Natalie now had three children so Mum got a lot of pleasure from the grand-children that she would never have had if it hadn't been for IVF.

She was a lively and active Granny to Cameron and would do all sorts of activities with him in the afternoon. Every now and then she would have stomach pains and we often blamed it on bugs being brought home from school by Cameron. Everyone with small children seems to be open to those kind of infections.

In fact unknown to us she had developed gallstones and these little episodes were biliary colic, intense stomach pain caused by the gallstones that would last for several hours then go. One weekend I went away with my mother-in-law Pat and other members of Wes's family to Dawlish on the South Coast and Mum did her usual duty looking after Cameron. We caught the train and on the Saturday I spoke to Mum and she said she had a bad stomach and thought it was a 24-hour bug but that Cameron was behaving himself. I rang again on the Sunday and she said her stomach pain was quite severe and she couldn't eat. On the Monday Wes picked Cameron up to take him to school and Mum said she was going back to bed as she still felt ill.

I arrived back in Bristol later that day and Mum had left a voicemail message on my mobile telephone while I had been travelling back on the train. She said she needed a doctor. I rushed round to see her that afternoon and called the doctor.

By early evening Natalie and her children and me and Cameron were at Mum's when the doctor arrived and examined Mum. He said there was no emergency but that Mum should go into hospital as he suspected she had a burst stomach ulcer.

The ambulance took hours to arrive and about 9pm Mum was taken to the Bristol Royal Infirmary. Her next door neighbour, Barbara, travelled with her in the ambulance while I followed in the car and she was admitted to hospital.

During her two days in hospital the infected gall bladder was diagnosed and she was discharged with some antibiotics to take. But she was in a lot of pain and soon re-admitted, this time for a week.

There was talk about her having an operation. My Mum was losing weight rapidly and then she was put on a "nil by mouth" regime to prepare her for the operation, but it was then decided she was not strong enough for the operation.

She returned home briefly again, this time with painkillers. It was clear to all of us that she was getting weaker and weaker and I got some special nourishment drinks from the doctor to try to build up her strength.

The country was preparing for a special four-day Bank Holiday to celebrate the Golden Jubilee of Queen Elizabeth II. Staging was being put up for a rock concert in The Mall in London and street parties were being planned all over the country. I was also due to go to a friend's wedding on the Saturday with Mum booked in to look after Cameron for the day. But there was no way she was going to be well enough to enjoy the national celebrations or do her duties as a Grandmother. The doctor came around to visit and pressed on her inflamed stomach and she vomited. The doctor said she was not happy for Mum to stay at home for the Bank Holiday and she was admitted to hospital once again. Sharon stepped in to look after Cameron so I could go to the wedding but all day my thoughts were with Mum and what might be happening with her.

That night her next door neighbour Barbara said she had been in to see Mum and the nurses had said her mind had started wandering.

On the final day of the Bank Holiday I went in to see Mum and she seemed a little happier and when I left she asked me to get some towels from her house. She was now in a room on her own as the hospital had a sickness bug. I left her at 3pm and drove to her house to pick up the towels so I had them ready to take in the next day.

At 2am the hospital rang to say Mum was being admitted to the Intensive Care Unit as her blood pressure had dropped and could I get into the hospital. Wes was working on the doors and managed to get a friend to come around to the house to sit with Cameron while I dashed into the hospital with Natalie and Sharon.

Mum was wired up to a machine that was at the bottom of her bed. She could feel the weight near her feet and kept asking who was sitting on the bottom of her bed. I signed the paperwork for her to have an emergency operation to remove the gallstones - something that I believe should have been done weeks earlier. Mum's final words to me as they prepared to take her down for the operation were: "Lou I want a fag". A lifetime of smoking had taken its toll on her but that was still her craving.

Natalie, me and Sharon were shown into a little room where there was a single bed and waited while Mum was in the operating theatre. After what seemed like a long while the surgeon came in with another person, we could see from their expressions that the news was not good.

I looked at Sharon and we both knew something was terribly wrong.

The surgeon said there was nothing they could do for Mum, her gallbladder had become septic and had cut off the blood supply to her bowel. He said that only machines were now keeping her alive but that after cleaning her up after the surgery we could go in and sit with her. It was devastating. We were in a complete state of shock. I was so upset I couldn't even call Wes - Sharon had to do it - and he joined us at the hospital as his work shift had now finished.

Mum was brought back from the operation on a life support machine and we sat around her. It was 6.30am. We sat there watching our Mum being kept alive only through the machines. We were a sorry crew: Sharon, the little girl she had rescued from the children's home; me, the girl she had created medical history in conceiving and Natalie, another medical miracle who she wanted after feeling she had to share me with the world.

There was nothing we could do. We chatted to her. We held her hand. Then we fell silent. We all realised there was no hope for Mum. There was not going to be a miracle today for the woman who had created the "miracle" baby. Older sister Sharon took charge and said what was in all of our minds. We all agreed that it was time to say goodbye to Mum. We asked the medical staff to switch off the machines and within two minutes our wonderful Mum slipped away.

Sharon and Natalie went outside for a much-needed cigarette and I sat for a while holding Mum's hand thinking about all she had gone through in her life and how determined she had been to bring me into the world.

Mum was pronounced dead by a doctor at 7am on June 6, 2012. Her death certificate said she died due to sepsis, an ischaemic bowel and cholecystitis. We came out of the hospital into the summer morning and realised it was too early to contact funeral directors and the other thousand-and-one things you need to do. So we went for an English breakfast in a cafe in North Street, Bedminster,

We trooped in having been awake most of the night and looking distressed and by chance we were served by a lady called Wendy Hudd. I knew her from the past as her husband had worked with Dad on the railway. We told her what had just happened and she gave us tea and sympathy.

While we were chatting to her she mentioned that she knew Sharon's sister Beverley and said Beverley would be upset to hear of Mum's death. Beverley, who had been adopted by a relative of Dad's as a little girl had dropped out of our lives altogether. I had never met her but it seemed she still lived in Bristol very close to us.

We kept Mum's death quiet from the media until her funeral a few weeks later as we didn't want press people turning up to photograph the coffin and turning that private moment into a public event.

The funeral was a quiet affair with family and friends and some people from the IVF community, including Mike Macnamee and Peter Brinsden from Bourn Hall Clinic. Mum had always been modest and never liked a fuss. A huge spread of food was laid out in her home and people stood around in the garden remembering Mum and telling stories about her. Martin Powell had a press release prepared and that afternoon released the news to the media.

A few emails sent from a small barn just outside Bristol prompted the interest and over the next few hours I watched on my phone as Twitter and Facebook and the internet went crazy with news of Mum's death. We saw it popping up in reports throughout Europe, across America, into Australia, India, Japan and national newspapers started running photographic tributes to Mum and her life.

I must admit some photographs popped up on the internet I had never seen before. The stream of tributes on Twitter were incredible with women all over the planet saying "thank you" to Mum for pioneering the technique that had enabled them to become mothers themselves.

Within hours it was the most read and most shared article on the BBC News website. Again the death at the young age of 64 of a modest, quiet lady who kept herself to herself in a little suburb of Bristol was somehow reverberating around the world.

The paper's carried a statement from a spokesperson for Professor Edwards that said: "Lesley was a devoted mum and grandmother and through her bravery and determination many millions of women have been given the chance to become mothers. She was a lovely gentle lady and we will all remember her with deep affection."

Professor Robert Winston, well-known on television and who has done a lot over the years to advance techniques in IVF paid tribute in the Guardian newspaper. Lord Winston praised the pioneering work of the doctors and scientists that had made my birth possible but said that often the role of the ordinary person was not appreciated.

He said: "What is often forgotten is the immense fortitude of the women who underwent this complex treatment, with repeated failure and agonising heartbreak. They too had extraordinary faith, suffering pain, repeated surgery, and the dreaded return of the next menstrual period when treatment was unsuccessful.

"Lesley, Louise's mother, who sadly died this week, was the first to have a successful live birth eventually and she was indomitable in persisting with a "hopeless "treatment. She was also immensely grateful to Steptoe for continuing to consider it, even when every option seemed pointless.

"One reason why Lesley and the other women were particularly courageous was because many experts argued that any baby born after IVF would be highly abnormal or die, as a result of this unproved experiment. It required resolve and considerable trust in Steptoe to face the prospect of a miscarried, deformed foetus, and worse to consider that an IVF baby might live briefly with a fatal defect."

Wise words from an eminent doctor and television personality but the internet also gave us the comfort of seeing tributes from thousands and thousands of ordinary people all over the world who commented on the bottom of stories about Mum's death or put something on Twitter or Facebook.

Mum was described as "brave and pioneering". People said she should be honoured. People said she had "enriched their lives forever".

It was touching. It was overwhelming. Of course there were also those who made comments about IVF being unnecessary and not natural. Even through her own quiet death Mum had sparked debate across the world.

One of the most amazing tributes came from Dr. Howard Jones, the American specialist who had been responsible for the first IVF baby in the USA, Elizabeth Carr. Amazingly, although over 100 years of age he wrote a whole paper on Mum along with Professor Eli Adashi, which was published in the journal of Human Fertility.

In it he said: "Oft forgotten in the ascent of IVF is the personal triumph of Mrs. Brown whose primary infertility remained unrequited for twelve long years and well through her 31st birthday". He outlines all the things Mum had to contend with to have me, not just the medical treatments and procedures but the emotional traumas and the press limelight.

He concludes: "Mrs. Brown did better than endure. She gracefully prevailed. And she did so in the face of a highly uncertain outcome… she placed her trust in medical science. And of course she placed her trust in Drs Steptoe and Edwards. Yes, Mrs. Brown was not the one to retrieve the egg or to nurture the developing embryo and engage in its transfer into the uterus. Still, her contributions of perseverance, courage and dignity were equally important and for that matter indispensable. Such is the power of conviction. In the process, a world has been transformed. The walking child-less in our midst are inconsolable no more."

My Mum…the quiet little lady who changed the world with her determination and courage. Life would never be the same again without her and the support she gave me. I was heartbroken. My sisters and I all paid our own tributes to her. We all had tattoos with Mum and Dad, written on them. Mine is on the inside of my wrist.

Chapter 14

SADNESS AND JOY

Early in 2013 I discovered I was pregnant again and it all progressed well with the scans revealing that it was going to be another boy - a brother for Cameron to play with.

Following a year tinged with such sadness with my Mum dying and Sharon diagnosed with cancer it was good to have a bit of positive news. But I also felt sad that this was a baby that Mum would never get to see. Of course, not to be outdone, Natalie announced she was also pregnant for the fourth time!

When we compared dates it looked as if we might actually both give birth at the same time! There had always been an element of competition between us but this was just crazy. Both our babies were due in August. Her due date within days of mine.

In April I got a telephone call I had been half expecting and half dreading for a long time. Bourn Hall rang to say that Professor Edwards had died peacefully in his sleep at the age of 87. The press, as usual, wanted a comment from me and all I could say was what I felt inside, it was like losing a grandfather.

I went to Bob's funeral with Martin Powell. I was a bit worried that there might be a journalist or photographer hanging around and they would notice I was pregnant. We stood outside the little church in the grounds of Cambridge University in the sunshine and so many people associated with my birth kept coming up to chat to me, saying how they knew Mum or had been involved in my birth in some way.

At the service those who worked with Bob paid tribute to him and talked about his socialist principles and how he had fought against so many critics to pioneer IVF. The words at the funeral brought home to me again just how important my birth had been to the world and just how much had been achieved by those pioneers Bob Edwards and Patrick Steptoe along with my Mum and Dad.

Bob Edwards had five daughters and 12 grandchildren and it was terribly moving when each walked from the back of the church in turn to place a single flower on his coffin. Then there was the poet Charlotte Higgins. She had been commissioned to write a poem about Bob Edwards for an IVF conference. It wasn't just the words she had written about the five million babies he had helped to bring into the world but the beautiful way she delivered it with her wonderful Irish accent. It was the most fitting tribute. This is the poem she read:

Five Million
In Honour of Professor Sir Bob Edwards

Imagine giving a couple who can't have children
the best gift they could ever imagine being given.
Imagine telling them that you can help them have a child
and give them all that brings,
give them family and hope, the important things -

Like perfect tiny hands and eyes that sparkle like cut glass
and inborn curiosity and soft skin
and 3am cries for bottle feeds and first words you can hear the world in

Like the stumbling wonder of first-time steps, growing into their personality,

and the babbling hours when they can't stop talking
the first time they come home from nursery

Like holding their hand on the first day of school
when their smile shines as bright as their shoes do

Like the lump in your throat when they head off to uni,
half-proud that they no longer need you that way

Like the very first date with the partner you know is the one that they'll
end up with
some day,
and the wedding day snaps as they both cut the cake and your mouth
and your eyes
and your heart smiled

Like the light in their eyes in the hospital room the first time that they
show you your grandchild.
Like having a child who is happy and healthy and yours, who is one
in a billion -

And now imagine telling that to not one couple - but five million.

Although the funeral was a very sad occasion it was also lovely to catch up with people I hadn't seen for a while, especially Bob's wife, Ruth, a remarkable woman. A scientist herself, she was the grand-daughter of Ernest Rutherford, who got a Nobel laureate in 1908 and then married a Nobel prize winner herself! I sat with her for a while and we chatted about life, my Mum, our families. It was the last time I met her as later that year, she also passed away. Bob and Ruth Edwards were an amazing couple.

On the way back to Bristol from the funeral we took a diversion to buy a baby carriage for the expected new arrival. I was so aware of this new life inside me about to be born. Somehow it made the work of those pioneers even more significant. Having babies myself, even though I never had to go through the trauma of IVF, brought home just how much it meant to people and why so many people wanted to know about me and my birth.

One night a few weeks later I got a telephone call about 9pm from Sharon and she said "I've got someone here who wants to speak to you." It was Beverley. Sharon had made contact with her sister following the breakfast discussion the morning Mum died, and they were together having a chat. We met up at Beverley's house in Bristol and I was surprised at just how much she looked like Sharon.

It was amazing to chat to her. We hit it off straight away and having lost a Mum and the equivalent of a grand-father in the last year it was strange to gain a new sister - one that was older than me. Beverley told us her story of growing up in Bristol. She had seen all about the "test-tube baby" in the media and had been told we had the same father. Apparently she had even come to see me when I was a baby. But things weren't good between Mum and Dad and her side of the family so she had watched my life from a few miles away.

Well actually, she revealed to me, it had sometimes been closer than that. When I was working at Asda in my teenage years she used to do her shopping there. She realised that the girl on the till was Louise Brown the test-tube baby - her half-sister - so apparently when she could she would make sure that she took her shopping to my till so that she could get a closer look at me and have a chat.

Amazingly, without knowing it I had chatted away to my own sister, helped her bag up her shopping and handed her change and her till receipt on many occasions without ever realising who she was. That first night together was not only fun for me but it was amazing for Sharon to meet her sister. Sharon was older than Beverley and could always remember cuddling her baby sister when she was little and how sad she had been when she had been taken away to the children's home, never to see her little baby sister again.

Her memories of that little baby had been what had made her so protective towards me when I was born and the amazing job she had done in being Mum and Dad's helper on all those trips abroad, protecting her sister against the demands of the media, the television producers and the just plain curious.

My life of twists and turns seemed to be twisting and turning faster than ever. Sharon's cancer had sadly been progressing and they had found secondary cancers in her lung, pelvis, hip and spine. They stepped up her treatment and she started to have chemotherapy.

I was now seven month's pregnant and went to Dawlish for a short break. Sharon was in hospital having her latest treatment and I called her on my mobile phone from outside the little clubhouse on the campsite to see how her latest chemotherapy session had worked out. She sounded pretty upbeat, although she said she was tired. I kept in touch with her by text and mobile all weekend but on the Monday morning, as we were returning to Bristol, I got no response to two text messages.

She had taken a real turn for the worse and when I went to see her in the hospital she appeared as if she had suffered a stroke.

On the Tuesday night - despite being heavily pregnant - I had booked tickets to see Mark Owen of Take That with my friend Kelly. He was playing at the O2 in Bristol, which is less than a mile from the hospital. We were in the queue outside waiting to go in when I got a call from Natalie to say that the hospital had rung to say Sharon was in a bad way.

I left the queue and met Wes and Natalie there. Here we were the same little group that had sat by Mum's bed less than a year ago - only this time Sharon was in the bed dying. She stabilised and doctors were confident we had not reached the end, so I went back to the concert. I kept my mobile phone on all the time in case I heard from the hospital and somehow it was better to be bopping away a few hundred yards down the road.

The concert ended and Kelly and I did our usual after-concert ritual of trying to spot Mark Owen leaving - something we had done as hardcore fans since we had been teenagers. We saw his car leave with him in it and Kelly gave chase in her car.

Here I was a seven months pregnant 32-year-old woman with a terminally ill sister in hospital and we were heading out of Bristol on the motorway in pursuit of Mark Owen. A couple of times we managed to pull alongside the car and have a look across at him.

We didn't really have a clue what we were doing. We were laughing and giggling like a couple of daft schoolchildren and we just kept going. Around 70 miles later his car pulled into Reading Services and went to the petrol station to refuel. We followed and jumped out of the car.

We dashed over to the car and the driver and Mark Owen were laughing, they had realised that we had been following them but they were a little shocked to realise we had followed all the way from Bristol. Kelly told Mark who I was and our connection of both being born in Oldham. It was a strange encounter with my heart-throb and we had our picture taken together and then Kelly and I headed back to Bristol.

Sharon survived another few days but we sat in that same hospital and watched her slip away. She had been another constant in my life. Her funeral was a jokey affair. She wanted *Bat Out Of Hell* by Meat Loaf to be played and she had always been a great lover of the drummer Animal from the Muppets so I had a tattoo with Animal on it as a tribute to my big sister, who had always been there. Of course I had another big sister now in Beverley. It was good that the two of them had met up before Sharon died but I was sad that they didn't have more time together.

It was strange for me in lots of ways to lose Sharon. I saw her every day as we worked for the same firm. So many deaths in a short period of time had hit me hard and here I was on the brink of bringing a new life into the world.

My second son was born in August, again by cesarean section. We gave him the first name Aiden, as it was a name both Wes and I liked, but gave him the middle names of Patrick Robert in tribute and memory of Patrick Steptoe and Bob Edwards. We knew that he had been conceived on December 9, my Dad's birthday and he looked amazingly like I did on the first pictures of me as a baby that went all around the world.

Natalie's new baby, born eight days before Aiden was called Aeron and when they were both just a few months old we took the two new babies along with our other children to Bourn Hall to plant a tree in memory of Mum. The worldwide media bandwagon was still following us around and both myself and Natalie gave interviews to the reporters who had gathered, including a Russian television journalist that had come along to talk about IVF.

As we tried to control the kids running around and get them to help put some soil around the tree for the photographers it occurred to me that I now have a role to play following the death of all four people that brought me into the world. I need to keep their memory alive and by just existing, I suppose I do that.

In Vitro Fertilisation has moved on incredibly in my lifetime and, although I am not a scientist, I am asked my opinion all the time about the changes that have come about. I don't really have too many strong opinions as I leave the science to the scientists.

In the early days there was an increase in the number of chemicals and pharmaceutical products used. I simply believe that if the doctors are honest and trustworthy and only use what is really needed to help people then these products are fine. Of course I think the more natural anything can be the better so we have to have in place rules to make sure people do not prescribe unnecessary pharmaceuticals to people just to make money.

Science should always be breaking new boundaries and if scientists can help people with the medicines and techniques they invent then that is surely what research and progress is all about. There are new techniques all the time.

I've been really impressed on what is happening with IVF and male infertility in recent years. That wasn't the issue with Mum and Dad at all but now there is so much being done to help men who have problems becoming a Dad. People's chances of having a baby, whether the problem is with the man or the woman, are now so much better than they have ever been.

In the early years there was a time where multiple births were a common result of IVF but almost by the day treatments are more sophisticated and that is a less common phenomena.

Freezing eggs and storing sperm has become commonplace helping people to have babies despite terrible life-changing illnesses and that has also got to be a good thing. Work with stem cells is helping to solve genetic problems before people are born.

The moral issues and dilemmas thrown up by my birth are still there, although the arguments have changed so much over the years. People's attitudes have changed incredibly and the laws have changed with them. It was unthinkable when I was born for gay couples to marry and have children. In the UK and many other countries of the world same sex marriages are legal and common and by using IVF, sperm donation or a surrogate mother those couples can complete their family with children.

I think it is fantastic that IVF techniques are being used to enable both male and female same sex couples to have babies if the children can be raised in a loving family.

IVF is also being used to help women have children later in life and that has been a mixed blessing.

Certainly it has helped a lot of women have careers and then have their first baby later in life, instead of feeling that they had to give up their jobs for their families. But I worry that it may go too far with so many women now having their first child when they are over 35.

More worrying for me is the number of Mums aged over 50 that are having their first babies through IVF. Although I would not stand in the way of any woman, any age, who wants to have a child I do believe that it is important that you are there for your children so I think people need to think twice about the age they will be when their children grow up.

I lost my Mum when I was in my 30s and I miss her every day. It brought home to me how important it is to have children when you are younger, if you possibly can.

The controversies continue and I'm often asked to comment by the media.

Early in 2015 the UK became the first country in the world to license the technique known as "three - parent IVF". It had been developed specifically to help women who carry severe mitochondrial disease have children without passing on devastating genetic disorders.

It means creating an embryo with genetic material from three parents. Opponents of the treatment have talked about it being a "slippery slope", saying it sets a precedent for the future and that once you allow techniques for altering the genetic material of an embryo before it is implanted back into the womb it is impossible to predict how these techniques might be used in the future. The fear is the production of "designer babies".

So many of the arguments I heard in the news while the issue was being debated sounded the same as those used when I was born. People always seem to paint a horrific view of the future when there is a new science breakthrough.

Of course society needs to work out how such breakthroughs affect moral issues, whether the laws over parenthood need to change as a result and just how far the medical geniuses should be allowed to go. Just as when I was born the rest of the world is following on from pioneering science in the UK.

Back in 1978 IVF was a strange science fiction process that seemed to be messing with the natural order of things. Today IVF is considered common-place and is an option for every childless couple in most communities, although in some parts of the world it is still a tough decision for them to take because of the moral issues and the cost.

The second I was born they called me "normal baby" and I try to lead a normal life despite the strange things that keep happening as a result of my extraordinary birth. Mum and Dad made world history when they created me - with a huge amount of help from two great minds.

I let all the arguments about right and wrong go on around me... all I know is that when I see my children and my sister's children I realise that IVF gives people more than just a baby, it creates a family.

A family that can live on long after you have gone.

HOW THIS BOOK CAME ABOUT

By Martin Powell

In 1978 I was a young journalist and I used to regularly meet up with friends for a drink in a South Bristol pub on Friday nights. One Friday there was a little fuss as a middle-aged man stood at the bar chatting to his friends. I was told he was John Brown, father of the world's first test-tube baby. Everyone was stretching their necks to have a look at a man who had been headline news in recent weeks.

Sensing a scoop I stood at the bar next to him and listened in. I didn't get much of a story as John Brown seemed a pretty regular person, just having a cosy chat. It was the only time I ever saw him.

A few years later as a journalist on the Evening Post in Bristol I heard tales of the Brown family that rarely co-operated with the media. In fact they would be positively rude if you went to talk to them and it was impossible to get anything interesting out of them.

So it was a bit of a shock when I got to know Lesley Brown and her daughter Louise. Lesley was a quietly determined woman with a good sense of humour and a loving nature. She was very careful about everything she said and actually quite shy.

It was clear from her personality that the last thing she would ever want in the world was to be in the spotlight. But the thing she most wanted in the world - children - could not be achieved without entering the spotlight in a big way.

By the time I knew her she had learned to live with that fame and realised that she could provide some hope and comfort for other women because of her place in history. Louise on the other hand has never known any different life. She is used to the media questions and takes it all in her stride.

The idea for this book came about after visiting Sofia in Bulgaria with Lesley and Louise and realising just how much their presence in a country they had never been to before could achieve. An ordinary Mum with her clerical worker daughter, who was also a wife and mother, treated as celebrities and meeting Government officials and eminent medical experts. It wasn't anything unusual to them, but it struck me that the real story of the test-tube baby had never been fully told.

Lesley provided all the information for the early chapters of this book, which were written in her lifetime. She read and approved the early chapters, which all happened before Louise's memory. When she died a remarkable archive of material was found in her wardrobe. She kept all the letters and articles about the family over the years and this assisted enormously in checking facts and details that otherwise would have been lost in the mists of time.

One envelope found in that wardrobe sums up the story of Louise more than anything else. It was from CNN, the biggest television news organisation in the USA, marked urgent in red capital letters. Inside, so pristine it could only have been pulled out of the envelope once and given a cursory glance is a letter begging Louise to give an interview. How many politicians and personalities would love to get such a letter? How unusual would such a thing be for most people?

But it wasn't the letter itself that summed up Louise's life. It was the fact that on the back was Louise's writing. That letter had sat in the kitchen for a while and Louise had written: "Mum. I'll see you at Asda. Lou".

A little glimpse of an ordinary girl putting an ordinary note to her Mum on the back of an annoying bit of mail that had arrived.